MEDICAL ETHICS
Bernard Häring

St Paul Publications

MEDICAL ETHICS
Bernard Häring

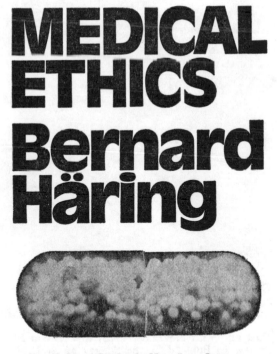

edited by Gabrielle L. Jean

ST PAUL PUBLICATIONS
SLOUGH   SL3 6BT   ENGLAND
Copyright © Bernard Häring 1972
Nihil obstat: G. E. Roberts
Imprimatur: + Charles Grant, Bishop of Northampton
            25 September 1972
First published November 1972; this edition May 1973
Printed in England by the Society of St Paul Slough
SBN 85439 087 1 Hardback   85439 093 6 Paperback

CONTENTS

PREFACE

About eight years ago the Society of St Paul asked me to write a book on Medical Ethics since the project was part of their programme and planning whereas for me it was an area of interest and of study.

In spite of my varied interests and many commitments, I never lost sight of this project. The work has been a challenge to systematic effort in this field, first, in view of the medical revolution of the past thirty years, and secondly in the light of new developments in the rethinking of Catholic moral theology, now better termed 'ecumenical ethics'. We no longer have all the answers; we are engaged in a demanding and enriching interdisciplinary dialogue.

My promise to the publishing house would probably never have been fulfilled without the most generous offer of Sister Gabrielle L. Jean, Ph.D., to spend her sabbatical year in collaboration on this task. The whole academic year 1970-1971 has been a most intense period of common work, research and writing. Sister Jean's scientific background in biology and psychology served not only in the editing of the English text but also in collecting, selecting and summarizing pertinent literature bearing on the contents of several chapters. The extensive bibliography is also her contribution. It is my delightful duty to express here my heartfelt gratitude to her.

We were greatly helped in our work by Mrs Claire Cauchon, Medical Librarian of Our Lady of Fatima Hospital in North Providence, Rhode Island. Mrs Cauchon patiently traced and retrieved literature generally inaccessible to non-medical persons and graciously met our every request for further documentation on a specified topic. I thank her sincerely for her very competent assistance.

The whole work was sustained by my assignment to teach a course on Medical Ethics at the Academia Alfonsiana in Rome, an institute for specialization in moral theology. During the same semester, I gave a few casual lectures and engaged in discussion with the medical faculty of the University of Bologna. I wish to express particular thanks to Signorina Anna Valentini, M.D., Assistant at the University of Bologna, who most carefully worked through the whole manuscript both from the medical standpoint and from the point of view of promoting interdisciplinary dialogue.

I am deeply appreciative of Dr James J. Scanlan's enlightened comments and suggestions. His insights as Director of College Health Services at Rhode Island College, Providence, Rhode Island, added a new dimension to the work. I should like to thank too Mr Wolfgang Goetze-Claren, M.D., for the lively interest with which he followed the whole development of the project.

B.H.

Rome
June, 1972

INTRODUCTION

The development of medical science and practice over the last twenty to thirty years can truly be called a revolution, and it seems that we are only at the beginning of a new age of astonishing inventions and achievements. As in any other scientific field, we can speak of the advent of a new epoch in medicine and in medical ethics. The many novel advances which underlie our unfolding knowledge about man and reveal the possibilities of his reshaping his very nature can be studied only in the total context of the new era into which humanity is now entering.

The history of medicine and medical ethics is best understood when set against the background of the total culture and *Weltanschauung*. A magical view produced the sorcerer, who also functioned as medicine man. With the sacred world-view of the Semitic and other cultures came the priest, who served simultaneously as physician. Ethical prophetism insisted, above all, on the relationship between human guilt and illness; its call to conversion held a promise of healing. Mysticism and esoteric religions of initiation afforded a symbiosis of ritualism and primitive psychotherapy.

The medicine and medical ethics of the school of Hippocrates would be inconceivable without the progress of the Greek philosophy of nature and the incipient 'desacralization' of illness and death, but it lived on and evolved in a world of profound religious beliefs. The confluence of Hippocratic medicine and the Stoic philosophic-ethical system led to another kind of 'sacralization,' that of nature (the *physis*).

The medical science and practice of the Middle Ages and the beginning of the modern era witnessed the conflict between the Semitic and Greek world views, between the ethical 'sacralization' of the given *physis* and a dawning awareness of man as responsible for himself over and beyond his physical trends. A further development was facilitated by the powerful impact of Aristotelianism on the medicine of the Arabs.

The insertion of modern medicine within the realm of the natural sciences is paralleled by the further 'desacralization' of nature and undoubtedly contributes greatly to this process. Man is not only coming to a greater knowledge of natural tendencies and laws but he is also learning to apply and to intercept them so as the better to serve suffering humanity. The modern physician is no longer hampered by any 'sacralization,' and does not hesitate to change a physical process whenever it is to benefit man; he believes that nature (the *physis*) is intended for man and not man for nature. We can call this principle the new 're-sacralization,' whereby the sanctity of the human person is the essential value to be served by medicine.

There is no doubt that by confining itself to the world-view of the natural sciences medical science has occasionally lapsed into a total 'desacralization' not only of nature but also of man. This is materialism, the most striking example of which is the pro-abortion movement supported by some physicians. On the other hand, we behold the fashioning of new myths: I think not only of certain Christian Science teachings and of the hope of redemption through LSD, but also of certain exaggerations of psychosomatic medicine and of Sigmund Freud's mythology of the *libido*.

Throughout this book, I shall repeatedly return to the real 'sacralization' which views the human person in the totality of his being before God, in his capacity to reciprocate love, in his existence in this world and in his responsibility for the world of man. I shall lean heavily on the anthropological medicine developed by men like Fourrier, von Gebsattel and Weizsaecker.[1]

Medical ethics tries to respond to the new challenges in a faithful awareness of the wealth of tradition but also in a sharpened consciousness of the newness of the situation, and of fresh insights, novel perspectives and increasing responsibilities for the future of man.

---

[1] Representative works would be: V. von Gebsattel, *Christentum und Humanismus* (Stuttgart, 1960). Viktor Weizsaecker, *Disseits und jenseits der Medizin* (Stuttgart, 1951).

B

Chapter 1

MEDICINE IN SELF-REFLECTION
AND INTERDISCIPLINARY DIALOGUE

The advances of modern medicine have greatly affected the whole of human life and continue to have a stupendous impact on it. Medicine and its prophylactic measures accompany the human person from the moment of conception to the hour of death. But that is not all. The progress of medical science and practice has contributed greatly to profound changes in the conditions of life, and the medicine of the future will probably wield even greater power.

In both its general and specialized aspects, medicine constantly accumulates more experience about man's being, body and spirit, about his nature, personhood and dependence on the world around him. It extends its professional interests to the relationship between man's environment and his bodily and psychological health or impairment.

So long as medicine restricted itself to symptomatic relief, to the treatment of specific organs and to the care of the individual person, it could eschew any radical assessment of its goal within the total context of human society. Even at that time, however, such limitation entailed great risks and had drawbacks. Today, it would be utterly impossible for the medical profession to refrain from self-reflection and interdisciplinary dialogue.

Contemporary medicine bears tremendous responsibility for man's meaning and total well-being. Such accountability arises from professional medicine's progress in prophylaxis, from improved social planning and from its being at the service of the whole nation, answerable even for developments the world over.

The case today is not one of moralists telling physicians about the need for self-reflection. Rather, auto-reflection stems from a general awareness and conviction that medical progress and responsibility oblige all members of the profession (especially those committed to progress) continuously to rethink medicine's purpose and to clarify its goal through sincere dialogue with the behavioural sciences, philosophy and theology. Throughout the past two hundred years, there has existed a danger that by basing itself one-sidedly on its own knowledge, methods and skills, medicine would develop its own anthropology or science of man. It sometimes tended to envisage man only from a diagnostic-prognostic angle and from that of the empirical sciences. In all fairness to medicine, however, it must be said that history attests to the fact that various behavioural sciences and even philosophy and theology often yielded to the same sort of temptation. But today, medical science is very much aware that it cannot isolate itself in its own tower.

The first great step towards diligent self-reflection was taken by anthropological medicine in its various branches, psychosomatic medicine and clinical psychology, for instance. Preventive medicine and social medicine pressed more and more for better structures in the family, society, the state and the Church, and called for more humane circumstances in the field of work. They demanded conditions of life that would allow the human person to protect his health or to regain it. The prophetic voice of physicians in relation to environmental pollution is but one of the many examples that come to mind. Modern prophylactic medicine is cognizant of the need to study the total physical, environmental, social and psychological context of human life.

Medicine is very much involved in an ongoing interdisciplinary dialogue on the most urgent problems of mankind. The medical profession expresses its concern not only about water and air pollution but also about the population explosion, the psychological effects of urban conglomeration (and more specifically life conditions in the slums), man's diminished capacity to bear suffering and eugenic-euthenic possibilities for the future of mankind.

With the shift from a one-sided therapy to preventive-planning, one detects a trend changing the focus of attention from the present to the future responsibility of medicine, a change from an individualistic personalism of the patient-doctor relationship to a social-collective accountability of the medical community to the whole of human society. There is a transition from the family doctor to the great medical team of doctors and paraprofessionals in the modern hospital and in medical research. This whole development is embedded in a cultural context passing from strong individualism to the present increasing socialization of life's experiences.

The very successes of medical science and treatment are creating some of the most perplexing problems confronting mankind today. The drastic reduction of infant mortality with the consequent rapidly increasing population in many parts of the world is but one of the great accomplishments offering new challenges. Another relevant but less glamorous and probably less studied advance is in the prolongation of the life of persons with a poor genetic heritage who, in past decades, would have succumbed much earlier to a natural death. Today, they can beget offspring and perpetuate the same faulty heritage, thus weakening humanity's genetic pool. So medicine today comes face-to-face with its newly-created problems and is now pondering on how it can react responsibly to the very undesirable side-effects of its triumphs. Medicine alone cannot bear the full burden of responsibility; of necessity, it must act in absolute solidarity with the other disciplines and with the *élite* of society and of the Church.

In the past, the doctor enjoyed extraordinary freedom in his self-chosen relationship with the families to whom he offered his services and who, in return, could honour him. Today in most countries medical assistance is socialized. The right to proper medical care is recognized as part-and-parcel of the most fundamental human rights. Such a situation leads inevitably to a socialization of the profession itself. The doctor is now only one of the many and various social workers serving in dependence on or in collaboration with insurance groups and social agencies. This is particularly true in the socialist countries of Eastern Europe and to a lesser degree in the Scandinavian countries, in England, and in practically the whole European continent. It will probably be so also for the rest of the world in the near future.

Doctors are a social force through their own professional associations and are willing to assume their responsibility in public decisions of the greatest consequence. Besides the problems already mentioned, namely, environmental pollution, the population explosion and eugenics, physicians have raised their voices on issues such as excessive smoking, drug addiction, alcoholism and particularly on a re-assessment of therapeutic interruptions of pregnancy. These are all problems of social significance and necessitate interdisciplinary dialogue, between medicine and jurisprudence, for instance.

Rapid progress in the pharmacological field, in mechanical devices and medical skills — to mention only antibiotics, virus research, organ transplantation, the promise of eugenic-genetic engineering and the new insights in biochemistry — has forced new questions upon us. For instance, where or when does human life begin? What is the moment of death? What are the limits in the manipulation of man? What kind of biochemical, pharmacological, surgical and psychological treatments affect the identity of the human person?

It is medicine itself or the community of physicians who, on their own initiative and under the compelling force of the new situation, have decided to interrogate the behavioural sciences, philosophy and theology. Such is the context in which we approach our task and the perspective in which medical ethics is set. Moralists are not imposing their questions on the medical profession, but are listening to its members in an effort to obtain from them as much information as possible, as both parties face the newness of the task in friendly dialogue.

In view of the awe-inspiring achievements of medicine and their impact on the total life of persons and communities, and because of our responsibility for the future of humanity, we are all confronted by the question of greatest importance: what is the meaning and the destiny of man? This inescapable but decisive question introduces a host of others: what, for example, are the limits to be set on the freedom of medical research, experimentation and planning? Morally speaking, what freedom does medicine or society enjoy in protecting eugenically defective life which may not only lead to the eugenic deterioration of mankind but eventually result in a substantial diminution of human freedom? We must also take into account the unhealthy forces of human agglomeration in congested, polluted and undesirable urban environments with their attendant psychological and social-pathological problems. What are the ethical considerations and principles that justify medicine and society's acceptance of these consequences as unavoidable? Or could it be that responsibility for the preservation of freedom obliges us all to counteract these consequences?

Obviously, in this sociological context, medical ethics cannot allow itself to operate within an individualistic framework of freedom. We are forced to take a courageous step towards an understanding of freedom expressed in terms of social responsibility for the whole of humanity and for the world environment, with a view to maximizing personal human freedom. We can truly say that here, too, we are facing a process of 'desacralization' in the sense that we do not cling to earlier modes of freedom as if they were 'sacred' or taboo. The new emphasis on freedom, however, which to me seems to be pivotal, can deteriorate unless we explore carefully its true meaning.

The way modern medicine handles biological trends, determinisms and laws affects the development or the stifling of human freedom. Scientific, technical and industrial progress has now attained mastery over these natural trends and biological laws; the consequences will be good or bad depending on whether or not responsible men deem it wise to react by planned counter-measures. What is the most appropriate and most effective course of action? What are the limits indicated and demanded by the sacredness of the human person?

It is ludicrous to expect the community of physicians or theologians alone to settle these questions. The whole of man-kind has to mobilize its intellectual resources and so structure a dialogue as to facilitate the finding of acceptable answers. The moralist will courageously but modestly insert himself into this ongoing dialogue. He can no longer be the man who has ready answers to all problems. It could well be that his contribution will lie in pointing to appropriate horizons or perspectives for the examination and weighing of contemporary medical prob-lems. Whenever respect for the dignity of man and his most basic rights are threatened, he has to raise a prophetic voice. If, however, he wants to be heard, he must show reserve in doubtful matters.

Knowledge of man: the basis of ethics

Knowledge of man is the basic presupposition of all moral discourse. It is on the great question of 'what is man?' that the moral theologian joins in dialogue with the behavioural sciences and medicine.

Today's theology centres fully on this fundamental question. That is why Karl Rahner calls his approach an 'anthropocentric' theology, although this should not be construed to mean that he sets man at the centre to the detriment of God. It means that God reveals himself and his sovereignty by manifesting his love to man, and that the whole of God's revelation tends towards man's salvation. A person cannot know and love the invisible God unless he knows and loves visible man. This is a theology springing from the dogma of the Incarnation which takes man absolutely seriously. If God reveals himself, his might and deity in all his works and words (Rom 1:20), it is that he wants to disclose his loving design for man and point to his destiny.

Theology therefore accepts the basic command of knowing God and striving towards an ever more perfect knowledge of man, in view of serving him better and helping him grow to a greater love of God and his fellowmen.

Such is the perspective of moral theology as it considers ethical problems in medicine. Moral theology cannot dispense with a continuous dialogue with the empirical and social sciences capable of promoting a better understanding of man and his behaviour. A more historically conscious moral theology is fully aware that knowledge bearing on man can never be perfect or complete. A historical orientation maintains a concept of man different from that of a static and self-sufficient theology. It is inclined to be less abstract, less individualistic, less conditioned by a fixed notion of man's intrinsic nature; on the contrary, it is more open to a dynamic view of man's development and his call to maturity, and is more aware of the great virtues of risk and courage. By the same token, it is realistically aware of the limitations of all human endeavour, knowledge and understanding.

Since the starting point of philosophical and theological ethics is the all-embracing vision of man, not one single science capable of contributing insights can be disregarded. Most relevant are the behavioural sciences of psychology, sociology and anthropology and the supportive disciplines of ethnology, comparative culture and even paleontology. By its very vocation, ethics is obliged to a continuous multidisciplinary dialogue. On this point, it meets with the best of medical science. Medicine itself becomes more and more aware of how confinement to the biochemical and physical world can be dangerous and impoverishing.

Both medicine and modern Christian ethics have learned a great deal from the phenomenological school of Edmund Husserl. Phenomenology tells us that all thought processes, particularly the formation of scientific concepts and systems, are characterized by typical reduction: the concepts are never the same as the total reality. However, if man is aware of this tendency to reductionism and its implications, he strives more consciously towards an integrated point of view. Humbly acknowledging this condition of science and of wisdom, he will keep himself open to the exigencies of interdisciplinary dialogue to complement his limited notions and theories. It follows that philosophical and theological ethics will no longer triumph as 'the queen of all sciences'. Instead, it will painstakingly study the methodology of the various sciences, review their findings and then work towards an integration of them all. This implies a constant openness and a readiness to revise one's own position and outlook without yielding to a despairing relativism.

It is particularly in the field of medical ethics that moral theology can capitalize on the phenomenological views already utilized by medical science. Beyond that, it has to learn from all schools of medicine, from medical practice, research and planning as well as from the questions arising in the process of research and discussion. The moralist surely enjoys the privilege of putting questions to medical experts, but it is imperative that he take seriously the problems and questions arising within the medical profession itself.

The pastoral constitution of the Second Vatican Council on *The Church in the Modern World* strongly emphasizes the autonomy of earthly affairs and science. 'If methodological investigation within every branch of learning is carried out in a genuinely scientific manner and in accord with moral norms, it never truly conflicts with faith. . . . Consequently, we cannot but deplore certain habits of mind, sometimes found too among Christians, which do not sufficiently attend to the rightful independence of science' (GS, Art 36).[1] The same constitution emphasizes likewise the need of a humble meeting of religion and modern science on current problems: 'In the face of these immense efforts which already preoccupy the whole human race, men raise numerous questions among themselves. What is the meaning and value of this feverish activity? How should all these things be used? To the achievement of what goals are the strivings of individuals and societies heading? The Church

---

[1] In a footnote to this article, there is reference to the Galileo case.

guards the heritage of God's Word and draws from it religious and moral principles, without always having at hand the solution to particular problems' (GS, Art 33).

Because of the broad scope of medicine (prophylactic, therapeutic, and planning for the future), medical scientists seek a holistic vision of man, particularly in view of eugenic possibilities and organ transplantation, which pose serious questions of immediate interest also to the moral theologian. The modern physician can no longer approach biological and medical decisions without being ready to raise fundamental human questions, and search for answers to them. The mandate is forced upon him by his position within today's society since the meaning of man's existence belongs to what is thematic in his own discipline.

It is within the framework of a pluralistic society and even within a pluralistic Christianity and Church that medicine initiates and carries on its dialogue. Fully conscious of this new situation, the Christian ethicist will no longer be content to quote past authorities, from Aristotle to St Thomas Aquinas, or encyclicals and discourses of earlier popes. There is no doubt that the moralist will always treasure past insights, experiences and endeavours; for he has much to learn from the magisterium and from the collected wisdom of his own discipline. If, however, he wishes to avoid all kinds of dichotomy and alienation, he has to participate realistically in the dialogue of contemporary man with modern medicine.

Some years ago, prior to Pope Paul's pronouncement in *Humanae Vitae,* a Catholic demographer told me that it would be wisest for the Catholic Church to cling to its past principles and formulations because demographic development would be unaffected by any new declaration emanating from Rome. This gentleman sincerely adhered to the teachings of *Casti Connubii* for his private conscience while, as a demographer, he remained totally untouched by it.

If I mention this example of a demographer, it is because a similar attitude can be found among some physicians and representatives of medical science. Their teaching reflects their concern with medicine solely as a natural science or with its technical possibilities, while their private life reveals a more humanistic and religious view of man. So there is a dichotomy in their convictions, a hiatus between their professional life and their private life.

The moralist can be similarly affected. If he clings to the old schemes of his discipline, to pre-scientific formulations and ancient philosophies (wrongly understood *philosophia perennis*) and if, in this attitude, he offers solutions to modern medical problems in the old idiom, he certainly does nothing to rid himself of schizoid tendencies.

For both the ethicist and the physician, the question cannot be limited to the meaning of illness; it pertains to the very meaning of the personal life of the sick or healthy man as well as to his fathoming the sense of illness when facing death. These are basic probings arising from the interdependence of illness and the finding of life's meaning, the relationship between the concept of the human person and the goals of medical science and practice. The burning questions relative to manipulation, man's right to dispose of his own organs, health and life, the bounds of the individual freedom of the patient and/or the physician, are all problems set in a social context and with an inescapable responsibility for mankind.

Medical ethics starts from the very questions which confront today's medical scientists and the whole of mankind, and collaborates with them in planning for the future. They are issues about which the medical profession questions itself seriously but which doctors shout into the ears of all who are co-responsible for the future of humanity. Having acknowledged the need for self-reflection and for a delimitation of its own task, medicine realizes further the urgency of an integrated outlook, and so constantly seeks a dynamic synthesis, one friendly to the process of learning and searching.

Chapter 2

THEOLOGY'S CONTRIBUTION
TO MEDICAL ETHICS

Although moralists are making an honest effort to enlighten themselves, the physician, the patient and all those interested in matters of health, they do not consider their prime contribution to be in the form of ready solutions. As indicated earlier, theology's task lies mainly in promoting a holistic view of man, and so helping medicine to meet the challenge of the times without being overwhelmed by neurotic anxiety.

This chapter merely attempts to summarize what revelation and theology's reflection on it can contribute towards an integral vision of man. The theoretical considerations advanced here will underpin the practical conclusions in subsequent chapters.

1. The dogma of creation by God who is love inspires man with profound respect for all created things, and grants him great freedom over whatever is less than the human person. Belief in *One God, Creator of all things,* is a call to co-responsibility.

Christian faith and theology centre in Christ through whom (the creative Word) and for whom (the incarnate Word) all things are made. As 'man for others' he reveals God's loving

11

design for us. To know Christ means to fathom the brotherhood of man in the fatherhood of God. It prevents man's alienation from God or from his neighbour by committing him to
worship the one heavenly Father while maintaining a vital
interest in the human affairs of the terrestrial community. We
discern Christ as the point Omega towards which the world's
evolution and the whole of human history are tending. If we
say that Christ is God's final Word to mankind, the statement
must not be construed to mean that after Christ's coming, man
grasps fully all the details of God's masterly plan; rather, in
the light of Christ, all new events, insights and endeavours
become a progressive revelation of God in time.

2.   The Incarnation establishes a new relationship between man
and the ongoing creation; it testifies to God's constant presence
to man through his work. God's handiwork addresses itself to
man; it is always a word or a gift to man, a challenge to openness, a call to selfless service of others as needs arise. By reason
of the creation of all things in God and redemption in Jesus
Christ, the Christian, more than any other man, is entrusted
with the task of cultivating the earth and refining his own
nature.

Revelation teaches man to consider his body in the totality
of his personal and communal existence. It disallows any separation of the material aspect from the spiritual, referring as it
does to the human person subsisting in a body, living in the
physical world in communion with his fellowmen and in
mysterious solidarity with the cosmos.

3.   Revelation has an eschatological orientation. While grate-
fully recollecting all past efforts, it calls for openness to the
here-and-now and for readiness in setting out for new horizons.
A *theologia viatorum*, a theology for the pilgrim situation of
man, inspires hope and demands responsibility for the future.
It summons to solidarity with all mankind. Modern medicine
has experienced how man's existence is affected by his environment. It therefore behooves all members of the professions which
take care of him to assume responsibility for the world around

them to the benefit of their own health and that of their fellowmen. Medical planning is unthinkable without opening on to this vista.

4. The concept of autonomy for the various sciences is very dear to modern theology. By its very nature, theology is indebted to and deeply appreciative of those sciences that contribute to a better and more comprehensive understanding of man, of his biochemical make-up, of his meaning and vocation. The distinctive and unique contribution of revelation is to assist man in his quest for the meaning of his human existence. It is only within this context that the autonomy of the various sciences can be redeemed from isolation and self-sufficiency.

5. The whole of theological medical ethics must evince a consciousness of the basic concepts of sin and redemption. Jesus repudiated the prevailing Semitic outlook that identified illness with sin, but he disclosed a marvellous *rapprochement* between redemption and healing, between redemption and liberation. Not only was Christ called the Redeemer, he was also called the Healer, the divine Physician. A belief in redemption impels one to attend to human health problems, both for the sake of the human person's integrity and for the sake of a social context which will encourage man's growth to the full stature of his dignity, liberty and balance. In other words, redemption is not a mere transcendental concept; our other-worldly hope includes the care of man in his pilgrim situation.

6. Professional ethics appeals to all those who, by research, science and/or practice, serve human health, and find in revelation a deeper understanding of their charism. They can learn how to steep all their activity in the love and justice which God revealed through his Son, Jesus Christ.

7. Revelation, and particularly the great prophetic tradition which reached its apex in Christ, has led to a liberating 'desacralization' of nature in its falsely mystified sense. The doctrine of the Incarnation and Redemption guarantees man (especially the physician) full freedom in the service of his

fellowman to the best of his ability without being hemmed in by taboos. It likewise safeguards the dignity of the human person in a perspective of the total vocation of man.

8. The passion-death-resurrection of Christ and faith in the resurrection of the body shed a unique light on man's bodily existence and on the meaning of illness, suffering and death. No other religion or philosophy has given so much consideration to the dignity of man's body; it is seen as a focal point for the visible manifestation of God's glory. In his body, man (and Christ in a unique way) is a tangible image of God. If this human body can experience deep suffering or be affected by an inauspicious heritage and unpropitious environment, it can also mediate and express the highest qualities of personhood: love, joy, peace, graciousness and gentleness. The body-spirit relationship and the attitude towards one's own body and that of others represent fundamental issues in theology. Here is a point where the existential and empirical knowledge of medicine meets with and complements the perspective provided by revelation. Biblical theology demonstrates that revelation, while profoundly enriching man's self-understanding, makes use of the world-view, the experiences and the philosophical outlook of a particular culture. The specifically Christian vision therefore has to take account, in continually changing situations, of the existential and scientific views of medicine relative to man's bodily existence.

Chapter 3

THE ETHOS OF THE ETHICIST
IN MODERN MEDICINE

Years ago I conducted a retreat for a group of judges and lawyers where we engaged in long discussions bearing on the conditions under which a lawyer could accept a divorce case. I explained at length the principles governing cooperation in sinful actions. Consequently, I tended to bar the lawyer's cooperation in all divorce cases that were not justified by the principles of Catholic moral theology.

One lawyer opposed me strongly and proceeded to expound the reasons why he accepted all cases that came to him. About eighty per cent of his divorce clientèle came after a bad weekend, in the first explosion of anger. The lawyer painstakingly explained to the divorce-seeking partners how to prepare the many documents required for processing the case. Each partner was constrained to work incessantly for a whole week in order to provide the basic documentation. Nine out of ten thereby came to their senses and gave up the idea of divorce. Others were helped emotionally and even morally in the course of the first weeks' meetings and discussions.

These lawyers were not merely following abstract theological principles about cooperation in sinful actions; they were render-

15

ing an altogether significant service to persons and couples who came to them. Theirs were not objective cases governed by one or two moral principles; they were persons to be helped. While juridical principles were not overlooked, they could never override the well-being of persons and families. By this and similar experiences I discovered much about the ethos of different professional groups, and I learned even more about what my own ethos as an ethicist should be.

In contemporary language, we distinguish between morality and ethos, between ethical principles and ethos. *Morality* is fundamentally the same for all men. Later on, I will discuss the plurality of ethical principles as a function of the plurality of cultures, but the basic principles of morality remain the same for all people at all times. *Ethical principles* are formulated in view of concrete problems and needs. The *ethos* characterizes a professional culture of morally-guided persons; it is worked out within the occupational group for the fulfilment of their professional task and vocation.

The ethos of the physician differs from the moral principles imposed upon him by philosophy, theology or his own Church. Each professional group develops its own ethos. Take, for example, the ethos of the policeman: characteristically, he defends order. The ethos of the politician is based on his dedication to the common good, to the best of his ability; with time, he accumulates extensive experience in the art of the possible.

The ethicist of the past, impelled by his very ethos, engaged in a kind of dialogue with various professional groups, but he functioned too much like a policeman, concerned as he was for defending the validity of his ethical principles. An ethicist is assuredly a man dedicated to the common good. Assuming that he is also a humanist and a Christian, he is a good listener, who can effectively promote significant dialogue, and speak a timely and forward-looking word to help towards discernment. He is not an isolated beam of light. If ideally he is in contact with the great ethical tradition, he also remains in touch with the contemporary community of ethicists and devoted to his Church or religious confessional group.

A moral theologian holds no monopoly in moral questions. Whenever he is called upon for enlightenment, he finds himself in the position of a learner, indebted to those who have particular experience in the field in question and have come to a highly developed ethos of their own. The ethicist should have learned from leading political scientists what it means to develop from within the best possible political ethos. Similarly, he should learn from the physician and all those dedicated to the care of health what kind of ethos they have developed and how, by themselves, they are working out an ethical code. The ethicist must always take into account the moral conscience and experience of those to whom he is directing his discourse. He has to conduct himself in a manner analogous to that of the magisterium of the Church, which cannot fulfil its function without attuning itself to the *sensus fidelium*, the experience of faith by the whole people of God.

From medical science, experience and competence, there emerge irreplaceable ethical insights. In the case of a specific ethos, if we speak on medical ethics and the ethos of today's physician, we must take into account the manifold branches, schools and trends within the whole medical profession, therapy for example, prophylaxis, planning or research.

The points I advance here are not intended to be a kind of ethical code for ethicists, but rather rudiments of the ethos which should characterize the professional ethicist active in the field of medical ethics.

1. The ethicist keeps abreast of medical advances and is sharply aware of how progress in both medical science and medical practice enriches the total knowledge of man and, consequently, ethical science. He will approach his task with the reserved attitude of the many great scientists and practitioners in medicine who humbly acknowledge the tentative nature of their efforts and cautiously indicate the degrees of certainty or doubt and the need for further study and reflection. This attitude will influence the ethos of ethicists whose particular profession is to reflect both on the ethos and on moral problems. A few examples may reveal the import of this comment.

(a) Medical progress underlines the tremendous importance of the cerebral cortex as the organic basis for responsible psychosomatic equilibrium. All questions pertaining to consciousness, identity, personal life, hominization and death must take into account what medical science provides as evidence in this field.

(b) The progress of psychiatry and clinical psychology has rid us of a great many mystifying ideas which became widespread even throughout Christian cultures — for instance, wrong judgments about mental illness, particularly epilepsy, superficial ideas about the relationship between sin and mental illness, and the whole collective witch-hunting that persecuted countless mentally deranged persons. In cases where relatives previously called for the exorcist, they now send the sick person to the psychiatrist. Some mental abnormalities and aberrations have been localized in the brain and may be minimized or corrected by pharmacological and other treatments.

(c) In innumerable instances, medical science has forced moralists to revise their concepts about guilt. Besides the insights afforded by psychoanalysis and clinical psychology, attention has been drawn to the chromosomal abnormality referred to as the XYY syndrome, which is linked with sex crimes and sociopathic tendencies. Young Speck of Chicago accused of murdering eight student nurses has recently pleaded innocent on the grounds of this faulty chromosomal packaging. Jurisprudence and moral theology are naturally interested in these new insights relative to the imputation of guilt.

(d) Extensive medical research has revealed a striking interdependence of behaviour and the hormonal economy. The prognostic value of the findings in this field justified the publication of a scientific journal devoted solely to this aspect of behaviour.[1] It gives rise to much soul-searching on the part of moralists who tended to pass easy judgments on people. At the same time, new fields of human responsibility follow on the heels of the better understanding.

---

[1] *Neuroendocrinology* (First volume appeared in 1965).

(e) The preservation and reproduction of living human cells gives a clearer picture of the genetic make-up of each person. The obvious consequences flowing from such a scientific break-through are many; for example, a priest or a moralist today cannot consider himself competent in those aspects of marriage counselling dealing with eugenics. On every team for marriage or premarital counselling, there should be a doctor who, fully aware of his personal limitations in this area, can properly refer to more competent colleagues in the field. The growing body of knowledge in this domain will give rise to many questions pertaining to eugenic responsibilities on both the personal and the social level.

2.   Moralists are certainly expected to take advantage of the expansion of knowledge enriching the whole of humanity; they should also keep informed about the problematic areas of all branches of the medical profession, of the technicians in the field, of the situation of the patient, and of the enormous complexity of modern health services and prophylactic possibilities. From this will follow a much more reserved attitude on the part of the ethicist who will still have to work out a casuistic typology. I am not implying that in similar cases he will arrive at dissimilar conclusions, but he will be inclined to state and apply a number of moral principles with greater reserve.

3.   The ethicist should know about the different training pro-grammes for physicians in various schools and countries. He will then appreciate the diversities of the medical ethos which arise from different specializations, different professional levels and a different *Weltanschaung*.

The ethicist cannot ignore the characteristic temptations (even institutionalized temptations) of the modern physician. In the countries where health has become equated with utility or productivity, economic and social concerns tend to prevail over personal well-being. The industrial physician catering to the institutional employer serves the interests of the firm rather better than those of the employee. The temptation is strong to clear a person as 'fit for work' where the same physician would have reservations or would definitely protract the return to work if the employee were his private patient.

4. It belongs to the ethos of the ethicist that, through his contacts with the world of physicians, he come to an ever keener awareness of the limits of his knowledge in his own discipline as well as in the field of the physician-partner. He reasons that many values and principles have to be taken into account before a concrete judgment can be made or any decision reached. This does not mean that he discards all the principles formulated earlier, but at this juncture of history it belongs to the ethos of the ethicist not only to revise this or that principle or solution, but to explore more appropriate approaches to the whole field. He assumes rightly that there are abiding moral principles which will inspire physicians to revise their ethical codes whenever they are faced with totally new insights and problems.

We moralists must not confuse matters of morality or concrete ethical codes with questions of policy and procedure. In fact, it is possible for a given policy or procedure to cancel out the ethical consideration on which it was presumed to be based. We are then justified in questioning it on ethical grounds, 'but we need to be careful about raising the cry of "unethical" short of such clearcut evidence'.[2] In matters pertaining to policy and procedures, such as determining the limits of reasonable risk, moralists can help very little: 'I think the less we moralists interfere the better in many cases'.[3]

5. The professional ethos of the Christian moralist in an era of 'desacralization' is best expressed by a quotation from the Bible: 'The Sabbath was made for man and not man for the Sabbath' (Mk 2.27).[4] When applied to medicine, this means that medical research and practice is for man and not man for

---

[2] Robert B. Reeves, 'The Ethics of Cardiac Transplantation in Man,' *Bulletin of the New York Academy of Medicine,* 45 (May, 1969), 406.
[3] Ibid., p. 410.
[4] Cf.: Mt 12:8; Lk 6:5.

medical research and practice; or, that principles of medical ethics are for man, not man for abstract moral principles.

At this point the moralist shares common ground with the physician of the Hippocratic tradition and comes even closer to the modern anthropological school of medicine. Moralists cannot blind themselves to the past 'sacralization' of the *physis*, of the biological trends and approximations that swayed both medicine and moral theology. Many taboos blocked medical care and research. On the other hand, the ethicist has to defend the abiding sacredness of the human person and of the common good, to the benefit of all persons. He must realize, however, that the application of this absolutely valid principle to concrete situations is anything but easy.

The important task of the moralist is to call attention to the total vocation of man including his responsibility throughout his earthly pilgrimage and his transcendent destiny. Neither the identity of the human person nor the totality of his relationships to the family, culture, professional world, society and cosmos can ever be overlooked. It is of the utmost importance in all this (for it belongs to the ethos of the moralist) that he should not introduce his views and position as coming from the outside; rather he is to refine them as they are incorporated and developed within the medical world. As much as possible his starting point will be what his partner is already aware of and seeks to validate.

6. From all that has been said above, it follows that the moralist himself, while pronouncing ethical judgments, must never lose sight of the historical process of the development and maturation of the person. The full meaning of being-a-person eludes whoever fails to comprehend human life as dynamic growth. Similarly, a medical intervention can be justly evaluated only when its meaning is pursued in the context of the patient's whole life and in the light of the physician's intention. An example may clarify this point.

In earlier years when the nature of organ transplants was still in the realm of discussion only, a number of Catholic moralists asserted that each partial act had first to be judged according to its own ethical significance. Whenever a mother donated a kidney in order to save the life of her daughter and enjoy a fuller family life, these ethicists focused on the extirpation of the organ and judged it as self-mutilation. They insisted that self-mutilation was always intrinsically and absolutely immoral. They maintained that it mattered little whether the kidney was ablated simply to be thrown away as rubbish or used to save the precious life of a beloved person. Such thinking gravely sins against the ethos of the ethicist because it neglects the essential meaning of a human action in the light of man's vocation to reciprocate love in the image of God. Well-intentioned as they were, these moralists were forgetting that the Sabbath is made for man and that no abstruse sacredness can stand in the way of the holiness of love.

Chapter 4

ETHOS, ETHICAL CODE AND THE
MORALITY OF THE PHYSICIAN

Over the past decades there has been much talk about the
loss of the ethos of the physician or of the imminent danger of
its loss. At the same time, the medical profession has engaged
more than ever before in discussions on ethical questions arising
in its field. In this chapter, I intend to elaborate a kind of
comprehensive outline of that which constitutes the abiding
ethos of the physician and its changing forms. I will point to
the relationship between the ethos and the ethical code, and
attention will be given to the morality of the conscientious
physician. Of necessity, only the most essential characteristics
can be touched upon.

A. *The differentiation of ethos, ethical code, medical
ethics and the morality of the physician*

It happens rather frequently that there is confusion in the
vocabulary involved, and so I wish to clarify what the basic
concepts mean to me and what they ordinarily represent in
today's language. The notions of ethos, ethical code, ethics and

morality should be clearly distinguished in spite of their inter-relatedness.

The *ethos* comprises those distinctive attitudes which characterize the culture of a professional group in so far as this occupational subculture fosters adherence to certain values and the acceptance of a specific hierarchy of values. We are accustomed to refer specifically to the ethos of the priest, of the physician, of the military officer, and of judges and lawyers who commit themselves to social values of the first order. If it is used at all significantly the term 'ethos' implies membership in a vocational group rendering an irreplaceable service to the community and dedicated to values other than those of financial gain. The ethos includes a definite tradition, a sharing in customs and common experiences, and commitment to a particular system of values. It originates within the profession and is formulated more particularly by those who typify it in an outstanding way, namely, those who, throughout history, have stood out as exemplars of the profession.

The ethos is to be distinguished from the *ethical code*, which consists of a studied effort to foster and guarantee the ethos, but is meant to go beyond it by, in the case of medicine, assuring to physicians, to patients and to the public, a professional standard of human relationships. No other professional community has elaborated an ethical code so early in its history and so universally as has the medical profession. The ethical code draws its vigour from the ethos which it wants to deepen and strengthen, but it goes beyond that. As distinct from medical ethics, the ethical code represents a concrete effort to ensure definite norms. It does not intend to lay down all the moral principles involved nor does it seek to develop a whole ethical system as does medical ethics. The ethical code of the physician has also to be distinguished from state legislation. The code serves more as a guide than as a control. It is, however, also used to warrant a minimum of ethical control by the medical associations, and it sometimes wards off the necessity for the state to legislate or to interfere in medical questions.

Medical ethics represents a systematic effort to illumine the ethos and to elaborate the perspectives and norms of the medical profession. Of course medical ethics has to take into account the existing ethos. It intends to strengthen the morality, the moral discernment and decisions of both the physician and the patient.

The *morality* of the physician lies in his subjective personal realization of the proper approach to his profession, his living the fullness of his ethos. It is the physician's capacity to act according to a well-informed conscience and to make concrete decisions with an upright attitude, and with insight and discernment.

B. *The traditional ethos and changing emphases*

The traditional ethos has abiding relevance, as in the case of the ethos of the priest. That of the physician encompasses enduring aspects and values but also changing forms of incarnation, for example, a modulation of certain values and duties. It is when these two aspects are not sufficiently distinguished that we hear an outcry that modern socialization, experimentation, organization and complexification are destroying the ethos of the physician. As in theology and philosophy, we have prudently to differentiate the lasting from the changing forms of expression.

At all times, it behooves the medical profession to serve the interests of the whole society by promoting those common convictions and structures of life that nurture the ideal ethos of the physician. This remains forever an unfinished task. A misguided romanticism that clings to earlier attainments — such as holding on to the past forms of independence and liberty for the physician or to particular doctor-patient rapports — is indeed nothing other than an alienation. A genuine ethos responds to specific needs and possibilities. Of necessity, the ethos includes a relationship to present opportunities (the *kairos*), with an eye to their inherent promises and temptations.

The ethos of the physician has invariably been characterized by an understanding of his vocation as service to his ailing neighbour, the sick man who needs him. The intention of earning a living cannot be excluded in his vocational choice, but it remains a secondary motive only. A mature person's choice of medicine as a career cannot be prompted by financial profits from someone else's illness. Yet a physician is entitled to a reasonable fee as a sign of social recognition and as a prerequisite for total dedication to his professional task without neglect of his family. The best of the medical ethos appeals to the physician not to make his services contingent on the patient's ability to remunerate him, since the poor have as much right to be helped as the rich. Besides, the ethos of the physician goes beyond the firm purpose of never harming his patient; he must offer a dedication which corresponds to and even surpasses the expected social honour and remuneration. A medical practice in conformity with the medical ethos requires that the physician, in all circumstances and to the best of his knowledge and ability, strive to alleviate the suffering of his patient and to heal him.

In view of the demands made on the profession, a constant effort to increase knowledge and skill through continuous education has become more and more a part of its ethos. As early as the time of Hippocrates, the ethos called for gratitude towards one's teachers and demanded responsibility towards the whole medical profession. It was a common saying, even then, that 'the physician is a friend of wisdom, a philosopher.' His professional activity impels him to acquire a formation which is deeply and widely humane; for he is called to unravel the sense of life, health, sickness and death.

Traditionally, the ethos of the physician has been characterized by a close personal relationship with the patient and his family. This was originally founded, as it is today, on mutual trust and responsibility, on absolute respect for the person, including, among other things, secrecy concerning family situations and confidential matters. The physician was a friend of the family and distinguished himself by a profound capacity for compassion and readiness to serve.

The altruism of the medical profession does not exclude the physician's deriving satisfaction from personal accomplishments, creative activity and social prestige provided this carries with it an ethical recognition of the services rendered to humanity by medical expertise. A medical ethos would be inconceivable without personal gratification in view of the achievements and weighty demands made on the profession in terms of personal responsibility, intuition and creative innovation.

C. *The ethos of the physician in view of the new situation*

Recent giant strides in medical science have emancipated the physician of today from countless limitations and 'impossibilities'. He has within his grasp knowledge, instruments, drugs, methods and procedures which, a century ago, went beyond the world of fancy. The impossible is gradually entering the realm of realization. As early as 1960, a noted historian of medicine referred to this evolution in the following striking terms: 'The physician of the second half of the twentieth century is unconsciously orientated in his attitude by the three following principles, which are pregnant with promise.

(a) In principle, there is *no deadly disease*. The fact that our rapidly improving therapeutic techniques cannot save a cancerous patient whose disease has reached its terminal stages of development is no proof that medical science will not be able to cure such an illness at some future time.

(b) In principle, there is *no inevitable disease*. No longer ago than the turn of the century, it was believed that a congenital and inherited disease was natural and unavoidable. Do not the perspectives opened up today by the experimental transmutation of the germ plasm outdate the dictum coined as late as 1929 that "crime is fate"?

(c) In principle, there is *no incurable disease*. The diseases which today are termed incurable will, in due time, sooner or later, be technically made curable'.[1]

All this shows plainly that in the last century and particularly since 1900, the image which the physician has formed of himself has been essentially transformed.

In view of the knowledge explosion, the inherited ethos of the physician compels him to learn constantly if he is to keep in touch with new professional achievements and scientific findings. This situation fosters an ethos which involves indefatigable research and sharing in new insights. The modern scientific ethos developed within the natural sciences invites the physician to admit humbly his own limitations. He should publish not only his obvious successes but also his partial failures, so as to call the attention of others to the necessity for further investigation.

Progress in modern medicine is unmistakably characterized by *specialization*. This new situation must necessarily witness the development of an ethos of teamwork and of mutual recognition; it demands a sharp awareness of the limits of one's own competence as well as a general knowledge of new possibilities. The competent physician of today often seeks the services of other specialists for his patients. More than in the past, this new situation can strengthen his sense of service to the whole community and that professional solidarity inherent in the medical ethos.

If the physician is to remain faithful to the best of his inherited ethos, he must constantly channel his interests into a broadening vision of man's total situation and vocation. He will thus insure himself against a loss of the sense of man's wholeness and of the centre of life.

In the modern hospital or clinic, the general practitioner and the specialist have a tremendous armamentarium at their disposal. The patient in need of a physical check-up is usually

---

[1] P. Lain Entralgo, 'Das Christentum und die medizinische Technik,' *Arzt und Christ*, 6 (1960), 137.

sent to a hospital where he is subjected to test after test and is led from one technologist to another, each with his own highly intricate apparatus. Unfortunately, it might appear that the equipment controls the specialist instead of the specialist the equipment. Add to all this the burden of an extremely complex bureaucracy with a host of appointees assiduously recording all the data in the patient's medical history and likewise reporting all his reactions while under observation.

A situation of this kind creates the need for a profound ethos among all those involved in the process. A conscious effort in this direction is imperative, but not all specialized branches and levels within the medical profession demand the same ethos. For instance, the nurse and the family doctor will, by the very nature of their activity, cultivate more immediately the traditional philanthropy. In some hospitals, it is a receptionist, a particular doctor or a nurse who guarantees that the patient will not be lost in the welter of specialists, technologists and apparatus. They help the patient to establish that personal relationship so necessary for an ambience of healing. Evidently new circumstances press for a more deliberate effort and sustained motivation in the development of an appropriate ethos.

The modern state and society have become increasingly sensitive to their duty to care for people's health both by prophylactic measures and by therapy. The medical profession itself has done much to alert the public to the fact that all men have a right to medical care. This marks a great step forward in comparison to earlier times when too many doctors with an all too good conscience devoted most of their time to the care of the wealthy. Though the new situation does demand laws, institutions and organization, some states are going too far in the direction of monopoly by forcing more and more of the medical domain to come under their direction.

Vast accumulations of funds invested in the economy (in the form of pensions, insurances and medicare) constitute beneficent establishments in favour of the socially underprivileged. But, in certain areas, the very structures set up for the medical assistance of the indigent have become an increasingly adverse

influence on the medical profession itself. By their very nature
and without ill-will on the part of anyone, these social institutions tend to shape men's minds and attitudes. The weight of
organization and the massive socio-economic power follow their
own inherent laws. Since the funds are part of the economic
structure, they are governed by the principle of profit and loss;
the funded agencies must be economically productive to be
maintained. As a consequence, the sick may readily become
objects of profitable calculation. The physician who works within
this framework is exposed to its impact.

The industrial doctor is equally vulnerable, owing to the
expectations of his employer, which can result in a constriction
of vision. For many employers, the responsibility for the health
of the employee means simply maintaining his capacity for
production. Only to the extent that efficiency experts inform
them of the relationship between psychological-physical well-
being and effectiveness at work will they extend their conceptual
frame of reference with respect to employee health plans, but
never beyond the efficiency-production aspect. A physician who
commits his time and activity exclusively in the realm of industry
will come to evaluate his work in terms of productivity. His goal
will then be to restore the full efficiency of the worker-patient.
As long as he is aware of this particular pitfall and seeks to serve
in other medical branches and on other levels, he is minimizing
the risk, but if he rests content to serve industry at the cost of
an impaired humanity, the consequences will be disastrous. The
medical profession would then come close to Hitler's Nazism;
with the cooperation of the doctors, Hitler eliminated hundreds
and thousands of sick persons because their productivity could
not be restored.

An anti-organizational bias, on the other hand, would not
be an appropriate response to the new situation. The individual
physician and the medical associations must strive for a happy
balance between organization and genuine personalism, encom-
passing both within the new needs. It follows that the development of the ethos depends more than ever on the whole
profession, which can better assess the motivation of its mem-

bers and offer insights or suggestions for corrective measures at all levels.

Another example may help to support this point. If a physician is living from insurance payments, meagre as they tend to be, he will have to handle a great number of cases day after day, so many in fact that little time will be left for a more satisfactory fulfilment of his vocation, namely, dealing with his patients on a more personal and professional level. His assembly-line delivery of health services will at times force him to overlook the total meaning of health. The individual physician, then, has to make a much more conscientious effort to sustain his medical ethos. In some cases at least, he will dispense medical care to his patients beyond what the insurance payments allow. It is a situation behind which the whole medical profession must rally to bring about a change.

Another aspect of modern insurance's disservice to the medical profession arises from the growing tendency towards mutual distrust between the insurance doctor and his patient. The very existence of what are sometimes called 'insurable symptoms' may induce a patient to turn to the physician not so much for a cure of his illness as for some material advantage. To so institutionalize distrust would be dealing a death-blow to the medical ethos. Actually, a similar danger arises in the case of the military doctor who is expected to minister to the needs of sick and wounded men for the main purpose of returning them to the battlefront as soon as possible. This problem can be resolved only by a combination of personal moral standards and appropriate structures and institutions.

Undoubtedly, modern techniques and organization have transformed in varying degrees many aspects of the situation in which the physician pursues his work, particularly with respect to a personal approach to his patients. The new organizational strategies support medical-scientific progress and practice but there lurks a threat to the traditional ideals of the profession. In my opinion, however, it would be false to speak of the medical ethos being undermined or destroyed, even though the new situation does demand deep reflection and a systematic

D

common effort. It calls for a new responsibility on the part of the patient, the individual physician, the whole medical profession and, indeed, the whole of society. A more conscious search for the inherent values and possibilities would help to transform dangers into challenges.

D. *Ethos versus ethical code*

The ethos of the physician arises from his ethical convictions and humanitarian vocation, from the historical testimony of outstanding realizations and examples of these, and it develops through the mutual support of the members of the profession. It tends naturally towards a formulated expression and constant communication.

The medical profession ranked among the first in expressing its ethos worthily and pledging members to it by vows, oaths and medical codes. The oath of Hippocrates has survived for two thousand four hundred years. Generations of doctors have made it their programme and their pledge.[2] In many universities today graduates of the medical schools still take the Oath of Hippocrates in its historical form, changing only the words 'Apollo' and 'Aesculapius' for the word *God*. A greater number of universities now use the Geneva Declaration approved by the World Medical Association (in September, 1948), which bases itself essentially on the Oath of Hippocrates. The text is as follows:

'At the time of being admitted as a member of the medical profession,

I solemnly pledge myself to consecrate my life to the service of humanity.

I will give to my teachers the respect and gratitude which is their due;

I will practise my profession with conscience and dignity;

---

[2] Cf.: 'Die ärztlichen Gelöbnisse,' *Arzt und Christ*, 8 (1962), 1-34.

the health of my patient will be my first consideration;

I will respect the secrets which are confided in me;

I will maintain by all means of my power, the honour of and the noble traditions of the medical profession;

My colleagues will be my brothers;

I will not permit considerations of religion, nationality, race, party politics or social standing to intervene between my duty and my patient;

I will maintain the utmost respect for human life, from the time of conception; even under threat, I will not use medical knowledge contrary to the laws of humanity.

I make these promises solemnly, freely and upon my honour.'

Most Communist countries use different formulations, but even there, the Hippocratic tradition remains visible.

Beyond the Hippocratic oath, the medical associations of various countries and regions have elaborated more detailed ethical codes. These are rules guiding physicians confronted with particular needs on the part of patients. As codes of professional behaviour, they provide guiding principles for the medical profession or particular medical bodies, and grant protection to the physician, and assurance to the patient and to the whole of society. A medical code has to be stringent since the physician deals with the health and life of man. At the same time it must be flexible enough to allow creative decisions to be made in extraordinary situations, and in response to new needs and advances.

Medicine cannot escape the influence of the *Zeitgeist*. Any change in the formulation of the medical code should be a constructive response to the spirit of the times. The contemporary guide to professional ethics should integrate the positive elements of the present historical situation while withstanding its dangers and threats.

An ethical code will remain ineffective unless it is founded on common convictions or can lead to and foster them. Hence the necessity of devising the medical code through an acceptable democratic process involving the profession and society at large. In cases where the state determines or devises a medical code through political organs alien to the medical profession and the needs of the patient, it is likely to be less appropriate and less effective than codes emanating decisively from medical associations. The last century attests to the fact that medical bodies have successfully forestalled the need for state legislation and control through their elaboration of an ethical code inclusive of appropriate disciplinary measures for its observance.

The profession as a whole expects individual members to abide by the ethical code and to feel co-responsible for its implementation. They will be taken to task if they neglect to form and to modify public opinion on medical issues. Should physicians be remiss on this point, they will fail to endorse the full support given them by the patient and by society, with the result that the code will be ineffective. The more the code is responsive to changes wrought by the transformation of society, to advances in pertinent scientific areas and to growth in moral convictions, the better is the prospect of its being observed.

The medical profession cannot uphold and promote its own ethos and social *rôle* without supporting the ethos of other professions and serving society by helping it to arrive at moral convictions. Physicians are expected to be responsive to the ethical challenges of the day, but many cannot be met by the medical profession alone.[3] The written ethical code contributes to the vital growth of the ethos and shared ethical convictions; it appeals for a sustained common effort for a better understanding and safeguarding of the human and moral values of the profession. It is precisely at this point that the medical ethos and ethical code desire the cooperation of humanist-ethicists, of the magisterium and of moral theologians, for enlightenment on how medical ethics should be formulated and applied.

------

[3] Dwight L. Wilbur, 'The Heritage of Hippocrates,' *Journal of the American Medical Association,* 208 (May, 1969), 841.

E. *The medical ethics of the Church and the conscience*
of the physician

The protection of people's health and adequate health care
are basic social concerns. Everyone must strive to reinforce his
fundamental ethical approach to health questions and to resolve
the problems that arise. The Church, more than any individual
or other corporate group, has serious obligations in this area.
How could she proclaim the message of salvation and command
an all-embracing love without an application on her part to all
that concerns essential questions of life, health and human
integrity? Salvation, the health of the person and a healthy
social situation are all intrinsically interwoven.

When I refer to the Church, I mean the whole people of
God in the full solidarity of all its members. Within this, the
teaching office of the Church (the magisterium) and moral
theologians have their special tasks, which can be fulfilled only
in continuous dialogue and cooperation with physicians and
other experts in related fields. It is because of so many mis-
givings that I insist repeatedly on this point: it is in this perspective of the solidarity of the people of God and the particular
competence of the physician that I speak of the ministry of the
magisterium and of theologians.

Whereas in legislation and broad planning for the protection
and promotion of health in the population the state has a subsi-
diary *rôle* in conjunction with medicine, the Church proffers
its effort at integration by presenting the basic perspectives,
principles and motives. While the magisterium normally speaks
only on urgent and distressing problems, moral theology never
relaxes its efforts at systematizing medical ethics through un-
broken dialogue with humanist-ethicists and physicians. Theology is based on the totality of revelation. It questions the
meaning of faith and its implications for a right understanding
of health, suffering and healing, and tries to draw conclusions
about the ethical vocation of all persons dedicated to the service
of health, particularly physicians.

The moral theologian acts as a mediator between the magisterium and medical field-workers. The theologian who only handed down solutions and applied the principles enunciated by the magisterium would be useless to the magisterium itself and would fail to get the ear of the physician. His *rôle* lies in listening to both and accepting the creative tensions which arise when one confronts the other.

It is in this context that reference is made to the relation between medical ethics and the physician's conscience. I am here considering the medical ethics which has its source in the teaching of the magisterium and the collective work of theologians.[4]

(a) The Christian physician feels conscience-bound to view his medical vocation and activity in the light of his faith, giving particular attention to the image of man as its meaning is worked out in the community of believers. Revelation itself gives only general contours; the Church has always sought an understanding of the nature of man and of his historical journey which will be more definitive because based on revelation. Christian anthropology is dynamic and open to personal development and reconsideration. The physician himself is a partner willing to listen and to share actively; he is involved in the common effort to distinguish what is permanent from what constitutes only changing aspects of our knowledge and values.

(b) The magisterium has the right and sometimes the duty to speak out on matters of faith and on moral problems. Faith is not an abstract doctrine or a philosophical system but a message of salvation attuned to and concerned for the concrete conditions of life. It is a light for man in his pilgrim situation.

Traditionally, theology has carefully defined dogma as a truth revealed by God and solemnly proclaimed as such by the Church. On the other hand, it offers specific guidance on how

---

[4] I greatly profited here from the article of Alois Müller, 'Die Selbsteinschätzung in des Arztes Begegnung mit kirchlicher Lehre,' *Arzt und Christ,* 14 (1968), 199-204.

to live according to faith. On questions of morality, the *rôle* of infallibility is limited to the enunciation of the most basic principles, to declaring, for instance, the fundamental right of man to life and prohibiting unjust killing. In moral matters not predicated by divine revelation but resulting from shared experience and co-reflection, the magisterium (especially in our critical times) cannot speak without giving its reasons and the pastoral meaning of its position. In the realm of purely natural morality, that is, natural law, the believer is bound to the extent that the directives manifest rational insights and reflect man's shared experience and co-reflection.

Since the magisterium speaks on the specific problems of a particular time and with the tools of a definite cultural period, the theologian must be a master of hermeneutics, that is, the art of exegesis in the light of the historical context, mindful always of the actual occasion on which the magisterium spoke and fully aware of the degree of certainty or probability. If an utterance of the magisterium is no longer in tune with new insights and the modern context, physicians and theologians have a joint obligation to look for better solutions and, if need be, to inform the magisterium of this. Moral theology has never finished its task; it finds itself in the never-ending situation of the learner, under such masters as competent physicians and the developing moral experience of the whole people of God.

(c) The final court is the conscience of the physician and/or that of the patient, taking fully into account the doctrine of the magisterium and the endeavours of theologians and other ethicists without which a doctor could not arrive at a thoroughly well-informed decision of conscience. Such a task of integration is not easy. Physicians and theologians have to look closely into the different levels of evidence and degrees of probability. In order to form his own judgment, the physician not only turns to theology but also considers the moral convictions and ethical behaviour of conscientious colleagues. This view finds confirmation in the doctrine of the Second Vatican Council. 'In fidelity to conscience, Christians are joined with the rest of men in the search for truth, and for the genuine solution to the numerous problems which arise in the life of individuals and from social relationships' (GS, Art 16). Insistence that the physician has to act according to his own conscience is not an easy way out but one that demands an untiring and loyal effort.

(d) Doctrine and information, important as they are, can never replace the physician's personal judgment or decision of conscience. This holds true for general convictions and particularly for personal decisions in specific situations. The physician cannot realistically expect a solution or a response from the official Church on every new problem. He needs only to consider the slight likelihood of the magisterium obtaining quickly all the information bearing on complex problems to realize its impracticability. 'Laymen should also know that it is generally the function of their well-formed Christian conscience to see that the divine law is inscribed in the life of the earthly city. From priests they may look for spiritual light and nourishment. Let the layman not imagine that his pastors are always such experts, that to every problem which arises, however complicated, they can readily give him a concrete solution, or even that such is their mission. Rather, enlightened by Christian wisdom and giving close attention to the teaching authority of the Church, let the layman take on his own distinctive *rôle*' (GS, Art 43). The physician is ultimately responsible for his own conscience before God. A mature understanding of the meaning and *rôle* of the magisterium will help him attain that freedom of spirit which will guard him from anguish or guilt when resolving a point of conflicting duties.

F. *The conscience of the physician versus the conscience of the patient*

The particular relationship existing between a physician and his patient imposes on the doctor, more than in any other profession save that of the priest, an obligation to respect to the utmost the conscience of the person with whom he is dealing.

In many cases, the onset of the illness and the prospect of healing are contingent on the total human situation, including the conscience of the sick person. Many decisions of the physician have a definitive impact on the future of the patient, who cannot renounce his personal responsibility in grave matters.

In order for the patient to make a decision with an informed conscience, the physician has to provide him with the necessary information. If the patient, owing to his age or condition, is unable to judge the suituation clearly, the physician has to give adequate information to those who bear responsibility for him. It is no easy task to delimit the duty of information, especially in cases where the psychological well-being of the ailing person would be adversely affected were he to receive full information. When the doctor has done his duty in discussing the prospect of success of a certain treatment or surgical intervention he will, after sufficient dialogue, abide by the decision of the patient or of those persons morally and legally responsible for him.

In some situations, the decision is difficult to accept. If, for instance, a fully-conscious adult patient refuses a blood transfusion in accordance with the teaching of his religious sect, the doctor will abide by the patient's request to let him die. If such a request is not stated explicitly, the doctor will prescribe the transfusion in an emergency situation without questioning; he is justified in assuming that a patient wants to be saved by the use of such an ordinary procedure especially if such a restriction has not been unequivocally imposed on the attending physician.

In the case of a child or a minor, the doctor normally does not need an explicit permission from the family, at least for a life-saving transfusion, and can act on the presupposition mentioned above. If, however, the family has definitively insisted that no blood transfusion be given, the physician will have to distinguish the moral from the legal aspect of the problem. Parents who proscribe a life-saving blood transfusion practically pronounce a death-sentence on their child; they base their decision on 'religious conviction' or, rather, prejudice. Most countries have legislation which then defends the fundamental right of the child and opposes the prejudice of the parents. Wherever there is no legislation, the doctor will also save the life of the child should it be possible. However, when legislation stipulates that the physician must follow the dictates of the family, he will not always be empowered to perform the transfusion.

The physician often finds himself in disagreement with his patient on some moral principle or its application. For example, a physician may be convinced that in a particular human situation, only sterilization can ensure reasonable health or life for the patient and stability for the family. The patient may consider sterilization absolutely immoral, in which case the physician will present to him his ethical arguments and the medical motives prompting the recommendation. But if, finally, the patient has a contrary conviction, the doctor is bound to respect it. Should a wife, for instance, be in such poor health as to be unable to grasp the full import of the situation, the consent of the husband suffices.

The physician has the duty to give his patient proper health care even if morally he disapproves of the life situation in which the patient contacted the illness. For example, he must attend to the venereal disease of his patient; he would hurt the patient by a moral judgment or by contempt expressed in the refusal of services. If, after obtaining a criminal abortion, a woman comes to a physician for professional assistance, he is duty-bound to help her. In due time, he may refer to a matter of conscience in so far as this is part of the healing process, or he may urge her, at the proper time, to cooperate in denouncing the criminal so as to avoid harm to other persons. The Christian physician models himself on Christ, who sought to heal and never to alienate the sinner. Apart from that, the doctor must remain in his proper domain and avoid all loveless moralizing.

Just as the doctor has to respect the patient's conscience, so does the patient incur the same obligation towards his physician. He should never request a treatment which he knows to be against his doctor's conscience. In some cases in which the physician has a well-informed and firm conviction of conscience that a certain treatment or intervention is both immoral and harmful to the patient's well-being, he should expose the facts clearly, including of course the medical and ethical aspects. No form of outside pressure, not even the love he bears the patient, can allow or oblige him to act against his own moral conviction. The argument that the patient will, regardless, obtain what he wants from a less competent physician can never justify an action which is against the physician's conscience.

Chapter 5

HUMAN NATURE AND THE UNDERSTANDING
OF MEDICINE

Scientific interest in the concept of 'nature' is genuine, but the physicist's definition of the term is likely to be different from that of the physiologist. The variety of connotations becomes a source of confusion for all. There is constant reference to nature in medicine and medical ethics but even there the meaning shifts. Conflicts spring from philosophy and theology; consequently, interdisciplinary dialogue can be jeopardized if close attention is not paid to the denotative meaning of 'nature'.

As this chapter will indicate, the issue is not restricted to terminology; different uses of the word often disclose totally different world-views. It would be impossible to write a medical ethics without clarifying the concept of 'nature', and without reflecting on the diverse ideologies concealed in the use of the word.

A. *'Nature': the crux of theology, philosophy, and medicine*

1. *The concept of nature in theology*

The word *nature* comes from the Latin 'nasci-natum' denoting what is given by birth or what is inborn; it refers to the dynamic principle directing the development of that which is innate. So nature can mean our eugenic or biological heritage tending towards growth and maturation. Actually, the use of the term in theology most often ignores the connotation of inherent finality. Theology, however, frequently refers to 'entelechy,' that is, the immanent agency regulating the vital processes of a being in view of the goal intended by God for a given organism or for the whole of creation.

Theology's use of the term 'nature,' especially in moral theology, is ambiguous. While the theology of the patristic age expressed in 'natura' God's original design for man and for the fullness of man's calling in creation and redemption, there has developed a totally different use of the word in modern theology, particularly since Matthias Scheeben. Scheeben introduces a sharp dichotomy between the natural and the supernatural, with 'natural' referring to whatever by necessity pertains to man in any possible order, while 'supernatural' refers to what is gratuitous on the part of God, a gift transcending man's essence and meaning. In this distinction between natural and supernatural, man seems to live naturally or according to his nature if he lives without grace. Hence, 'nature' is an abstract concept, and a theology of it is a theology of possible or impossible things.

Good theology has consistently taught that there is one historical order of salvation and that man, where he renders himself inaccessible to grace, does not live according to a pure nature but rather opts for a disturbed nature. We can say that historical man without grace lives in 'un-nature,' in unregenerate nature. But this is not to deny the theological concern behind the proposed distinction of nature and supernature; this distinction expresses forcefully that salvation is a totally undeserved gift of God.

Salvation by faith becomes more visible where man, in gratitude, fully acknowledges that the actual order of salvation is beyond what any creature could ever claim or effect by itself. Salvation summons to adoring gratefulness for everything, and most specifically for adoption as children of God. 'Un-nature,'

or loss of salvation, takes over where man posits himself
as the centre of life and makes arrogant claims before God.
Un-nature assumes control whenever man becomes oblivious of
the undeserved goodness of God and of the loftiness of his
vocation.

Moral theology occasionally refers to 'nature' in a context
reflecting philosophical and modern medical influences. To some
extent this can be considered as normal (one is tempted to say
'natural') since moral theology has to express its principles within
a given *Weltanschauung* and with a vocabulary intelligible to its
intended interlocutors. A danger arises where theology is unwary
of the pitfalls of a certain philosophy of nature. Precarious situations have arisen historically from the fact that theology, while
explaining earlier documents of the magisterium and the
theological tradition, did not resort sufficiently to hermeneutics.
It failed to look closely enough at the connotation of critical
words in the world-view of that historical situation.

Within a static order of human affairs and an unchangeable
world-view, the concept of 'nature' remains unaltered in so far
as it seeks to express the *essence* of man. This applies to great
parts of theology in spite of the Bible's dynamic vision of the
history of salvation. An evolving situation that incorporates a
changing world-view results in correlative revisions of the whole
concept of nature.

It is customary for theology to embed its understanding of
human nature in a historical context, especially through a clarifi-
cation of the traditional and time-honoured concepts: 'natura
originalis' (original nature), 'natura lapsa' (fallen nature) and
'natura lapsa et reparata' (fallen and redeemed nature). Most
theological traditions considered man's original nature as given
historical realization at the very beginning or at the instant of
man's creation; they were most 'knowledgeable' about the preter-
natural privileges of Adam and Eve, about the perfection of their
intelligence and affectivity, their absolute psychosomatic equilibrium and physical immortality. Paleontologists and biologists
have since expanded our knowledge through their well-founded
theories of cosmic evolution and gradual hominization; many

theologians now assign a new meaning to the 'natura originalis,' namely, the original design of God with all its potential dynamism. It intimates what nature and human history could have been if, in all phases of development, mankind had been faithful to the call of grace and had responded by availing itself of all the gifts of God. We can no longer ignore the substantial difference in theological outlook between an ethicist subscribing to man's original nature as static and fully realized and one subscribing to a dynamic design.

At any rate, theology never exclusively endorsed static expressions; it definitively admitted a dynamic element when it spoke of the fallen and redeemed nature of man and thereby accepted a powerful tension component into the heretofore historical human nature. The fallen or ungraced nature is not to be confused with a 'pure nature,' since God never left man without hope but always offered him a covenant of love. When man refused God's gracious advances, he enfeebled himself and sought to avert his true destiny; he eventually decayed. A strong differential in tension-potential comes to distinguish those individuals and communities who succumb to unredeemed egotism and those who gradually and visibly open themselves to redemption in grateful response to God's benevolence and in unselfish love towards their neighbours. But the very fact that we experience the opposing forces of a disturbed and a redeemed nature makes it extremely difficult to decipher God's will as written in the given nature.

Today's theology pays greater attention to the biblical account of creation where, at the beginning, there was only chaos which gradually yielded to a magnificent order of things. That God entrusted nature to man reveals his intention that man, as an adorer and a loving being, overcome the chaotic tendencies in the world around him. Medicine, then, can envisage its task as that of subduing the disorderly powers of human 'nature' in view of the most desirable redeemed order.

The biblical perspective of creation makes it possible for theology to meet with modern man who, to some extent, considers himself as 'his own self-creator, for in a sense man is unfinished and capable now of creating himself.[1] Of course, theology must be alert to the danger of man's turning a deaf ear to God's expressed design by wanting to be *independently* his self-creator. Theologically speaking, this would mean that man chose to seek his self, his true 'nature' by existentially separating himself from the very Truth that gives him life. Man can find his true nature only by going back to the source of life. In his limited realm, then, man can share in God's creativity.

2. *The concept of nature in philosophy*

Each philosophical system has made a courageous attempt to define or to describe human nature; philosophical interest concerns the essence, the goal and the direction of man. Since one of philosophy's tasks is to reflect on the nature of being, it sometimes sees man only as a part of the total substance of the world. In philosophy, more than in theology, the word 'nature' reflects diverse world-views. The concept of nature in a modern materialistic world-view differs markedly from that of the Greek philosophy of nature which took the *physis*, the general nature of being, as a starting point. Different again is Hindu philosophy, which combined efforts towards personalism with animistic traditions and saw souls everywhere, in all things. The discourse on 'nature' in the explicitly personalistic philosophy of men like Ferdinand Ebner and Martin Buber endows the 'nature' of the human person with the constitutive relationship of Thou-We-I. There, man's nature or essence is distinctly and totally linked to God's calling, to man's response in personalizing relationships with his fellowmen, and to his ordering of them to the health and the development of all persons.

The 'natura rationalis' defines the nature of man in the philosophical tradition from Aristotle to Thomas Aquinas. This school of philosophy asserts that it belongs to man's essence to

---

[1] Charles Curran, 'Moral Theology and Genetics,' *Cross Currents*, XX (Winter, 1970), 73.

have a conscious life, to be able to reflect on his own being with rational concepts and to communicate with others in symbols and ideas. In much of Greek philosophy, the concept 'nature' is somehow linked to pantheism or at least to a pantheistic-biologic conception of God's presence in all living things. From the tradition stretching from Aristotle to the philosophy and ethics of the Stoics, which influenced many of the great medical traditions up to the encyclical *Casti Connubii* of Pius XI, we inherit the classical expression: 'Deus et natura nihil faciunt frustra.' Aristotle enlisted many followers with this teaching that 'God and nature do nothing in vain.' From Aristotle the dictum passed down through the philosophy and medicine of the Arabs, although the meaning of the combination 'God and nature' shaded into different colours.

The philosophy of Plato and Plotinus considers the nature of man almost exclusively in his immortal soul and its connaturality to a sphere of lofty ideals, in the *eros* that soars above the visible world including the body. In the philosophy underpinning the theology of St Augustine and the Franciscan school, the 'nature of man' rests mainly in his capacity to reciprocate love. This philosophical position also shares the Thomistic view that rationality, intellect, affectivity and passions belong to man's nature. But that which, in the Augustinian and Franciscan tradition, gives final meaning to man's being is the capacity to love and to discern genuine love from all its counterfeits. In Thomism, the unifying element is man's rationality.

Parmenides envisages the whole world, especially the realm of concepts and principles, as static. He stresses the identity of principles, ideals, ideas and essences. Heraclitus perceives everything in the perspective of becoming; man's nature is being in becoming, and the process unfolds in a world that is more becoming than being. Running through most of the Greek philosophers' views of man and his nature is a cyclic understanding of time, that is, the notion that in due time, everything will return accurately to what it was in earlier whirls or centuries. So both the static and the dynamic concept of 'nature' are set in a totally different world-view from that of our Christian

E

notion of man's historical nature, that is, of man in the unique and irreversible history of salvation.

Today's philosophy, from Martin Heidegger to Marcuse, centres the whole system on becoming. Nature is being by becoming. The courage-to-be implies the audacity to change and to accept challenges which are always new. At the heart of this philosophy lies the creative tension between essence and existence, but existence is often given greater value than essence. The inclination is strongly towards describing the 'nature of man' through the polar tensions. Here, then, the biblical concept of original chaos takes a totally different direction, as if man in his innermost being or nature would somehow be engaged in the struggle between chaos and order.

Today's best philosophy stresses the difference between man's nature and culture. In this vision, nature is the material for culture. It then belongs to the essence of the human person (or if you wish, to man's nature) and to that of mankind to be a wise steward of nature's goods including his own biochemical heritage and the fabric of his subconscious-unconscious life.

3. *The concept of nature in medicine*

Medicine and medical ethics somehow participate in the various efforts to learn about human nature, but as in theology and philosophy, their direction is profoundly affected by the *Zeitgeist* and the prevailing world-view. Vastly different will be the medicine operating with the mental tools of the Greek philosophies of nature and that using the modern personalistic instrumentation of existentialists like Viktor Frankl.

Admittedly, the methodological inquiry of medicine contrasts with that of philosophy. The physician approaches man in a much more existential way. He serves a real person suffering from poor health and so is not given primarily to philosophical ruminations on the essence of man. He is fascinated not so much by abstract ideas pertaining to man's nature, health or illness, as by his day-to-day encounters with more or less healthy persons. Consequently, the door to his knowledge, wisdom and skills opens in an existential sense with his intention to heal or to help suffering man. Since his thinking is inevitably linked to practice, he seeks verification of knowledge.

While physicians of the 'classical' school of natural sciences (in the nineteenth century) generally limited their efforts to the biochemical world, doctors like Weizsaecker and Frankl approach man, and specifically his neuroses, within a personalistic frame of reference. Their holistic basis of operation accounts for their taking seriously man's existence as body and spirit.

The concept of man's nature in the thought and practice of the physician necessarily emerges from the bodily existence of man, since the medical profession is historically turned to the curing of illnesses which manifest themselves in the body. Only within ancient religions where medicine was wedded to the priestly and prophetic function were sickness and sin so strongly identified that the body could somehow be neglected. The medicine man tried to exorcise demons, whereas the modern physician focuses his attention on man's total being in all the dimensions of his life and experience and in the context of whatever influences him.

In the great medical tradition, human nature is considered above all as the principle of life, of growth, of development, of man's inborn healing powers. The inherent dynamic plan governing unfolding processes is now better understood through the contribution of embryology. Altogether it can be said that the questions pertaining to the concept and reality of man's nature as a basis for medical-ethical norms plead for a profound understanding of man's existence in his body.

B. *The concept of the human body and the embodied spirit*

In some religions and philosophies it seemed possible to search for the nature and destiny of man by concentrating totally or one-sidedly on the immaterial soul; there was reluctance to accept the human body as truly belonging to the nature of man. For Christians, the importance and dignity of the body

is paramount, ordained as it is to become more and more a
visible image of God's goodness, mercy and purity. The man
who lives according to God's intention glorifies his Creator and
Redeemer in his body. We can even say that the zenith of God's
masterly design was his Son's assuming a human body: 'And
the Word became flesh' (Jn 1:14). In modern language, we
would say: 'The Word of God became a live human body.'
The wording of the Bible is the strongest possible expression of
the sum and substance of bodily existence.

The letter to the Hebrews epitomizes the beginning of the
conscious life of the Word Incarnate in the following prayer:
'But thou hast prepared a body for me . . . Here I am . . . I
have come, O God, to do thy will' (Heb 10: 5-7). In this context,
body means practically the same as human nature. As Christians,
we broach the question of human nature in the light of the
dogma of the incarnation and of the resurrection of Christ. A
spiritualistic outlook evincing contempt for the body opposes
itself radically to Christian belief. Even though the body is
tainted by sinfulness, one cannot consider the body alone as
source or site of sin, as if an innocent soul were imprisoned in
a sinful body. The Christian vision is directed towards man in
his wholeness. The whole man has his origin in God; the whole
man falls into the stream of sinfulness and is subjected to the
vanity of sin. So also is the whole man redeemed and called to
holiness, able to conquer the powers of sin.

Traditionally, the Christian doctrine of man's nature states
that man is a composite of body and soul or body and spirit,
but one cannot construe additivity. It would be inaccurate to
say that man *has* a body. Man is an embodied spirit; he *is* a
live body. The nature of man is not limited to a mere summation
of biological and personal characteristics; human existence on
earth is truly biological and wholly personal in the sense that
these two aspects pertain to the same reality and not to separate
parts. The consciousness, the deepest insights and expressions
of the spiritual person are never possible without the con-
currence of the body, most specifically, without cerebral-cortical
activity.

One of the greatest threats posed to modern medicine came from the theoretical medicine taught in so many medical schools which adhered almost exclusively to the natural scientific methods with attention given solely to the biochemical world. The danger of one-sidedness today lies in pursuing uniquely the analysis of man's psyche. In no way do I intend to deprecate a thorough study of biochemistry, but in medicine the physician must be fully aware that he is studying the biochemical reactions of a *person*. The theoretical medicine of many schools tended to fragment man by concentrating on the study of cells, organs and functions while neglecting the wholeness of the body which is the embodied person. In his practice, the physician meets either persons or corpses, that is, persons existing in a body or the remaining aggregation of quickly decomposing organs and cells. The true human nature to which the physician dedicates himself in scientific service is a marvellous unity of bodily and spiritual dimensions. Each of them will be better understood if medicine is fully aware that it is studying not a discrete part but only a dimension of the whole.

The specific nature of man lies in his being in the body and in being through his bodily existence open to the Other, to the 'we' of community and to the world around him. It is an openness of the whole person in and through the body. Man's body is not a thing but an embodied word, a message and an appeal. In his bodily existence man, like animals, craves subsistence in growth, but he is not content to remain at that level; he longs for love, understanding, community. The animal is not without a certain openness to the world around him which, at times, is a source of wonder for man; however, the animal's reaction differs from man's responsiveness. A startled animal can hardly be compared to a man filled with admiration and adoration.

Man is primarily distinguished by consciousness which predicates a centre of personality in relation with other persons and in relatedness to the world around him, a world transcending utility. He is searching for meaning and assumes responsibility for the fashioning of the world to the advantage of man and human relations. To some extent, the animal is more open to environmental influences than man; it instinctively adapts itself. Transferred to a new environment or subjected to new climatic conditions, if it survives at all it ordinarily adjusts itself in its whole biochemical and physical condition and within a relatively short period of time. Man is much less flexible in his physiology. He adapts to his world in a totally different way, through inventiveness and culture. Whereas the animal finds biological compensations, man as a tool-maker adjusts through invention and artificial means, although throughout the ages considerable biological transformations of man's nature have resulted.

The medical science of the last decades has contributed notably to an understanding of the wholeness of human nature in its bodily and spiritual interactions. Man's every act of consciousness, of reflection or decision, involves psychosomatic activity. Like the electronic mechanical brains with countless electrical currents and connections,[2] man's intricate bodily innervation can receive and send out messages from different cortical centres. An almost incredible wealth of information is stored through the heritage of generations and communicated through the genetic code. This, moreover, is the prodigious result of all the activity of a lifetime, containing man's communication with his fellowmen and with the world about him.

Psychic or spiritual activities, even of moral and religious quality, are not simply recorded in stored information and innumerable computer circuits; they merge into a marvellous unity. The most highly developed mechanical brain can operate only with the information already stored by its programmer, but man's creative power can unfold ever new possibilities. He can consciously take positions and make decisions. He has a way of feeling and acting which brings him into conscious contact with values and truths. The mechanical brain can be programmed to 'say prayers,' but it can never pray, nor can it share loving concern; it can never adore, nor will it

---

[2] Wolf Rohrer, *Ist der Mensch konstruierbar?* (Munich: Verlag Ars Sacra, 1966).

ever know sacrificial love. Only man can bestow himself freely in love. It could well be that the computer can imitate some people falling 'in and out of love,' since their situation would meet the requirements of binary circuitry, but this does not compare with 'love' which is man's distinct vocation.

The psychiatric understanding of neurosis and psycho-therapy, especially in the school of psychosomatic medicine, has pinpointed man's 'nature' in terms of his body-spirit unity. Medieval medicine and philosophy asserted that the soul could never become sick. All the psychopathologies were therefore conveniently shunted into somatic disturbances unless one chose to explain them by demonic forces. Modern medicine knows more of the amazing correlations between somatic distress and psychopathology; ailments that are not organic have at least a somatic resonance. Emphasis on this fact resulted in a healthy reaction by medical scholars against the trend towards extreme psychopathology and psychotherapy that insisted exclusively on the psychogenic element and often neglected the patient's body. More than ever today, modern medicine realizes the need for a physician to attend to both dimensions.

C. *Is there a nature in which we can read God's will?*

The question of whether God's will is readably written in nature must be studied in the light of the diverse concepts of nature found in philosophy, theology and medicine. The history of medicine and of culture serves as a caution against any oversimplification. A constant quest for an improved understand-ing of man's nature will lead to a better comprehension of our responsibility and of the full import of morality. It will then be easier to discern God's will.

Contemporary science and the modern world-view yield many new insights and perspectives which were not only unavailable earlier but were even unthinkable. For instance, we see that even in the physical world, nature is not as thoroughly determined as classical physics had led us to believe. The quantum theory of Max Planck reveals the tremendous relevance of those minimal oscillations which completely eluded the deterministic thinking of earlier physicists. The whole 'nature' of the universe now draws our attention to those cosmological leaps without which the evolution of the world and hominization would remain pure conjectures.

A medicine totally turned to the biochemical world or to a purely somatic understanding of health and illness could, with the old tools of Hippocratic medicine and the natural sciences, constrict medical rules and procedures by attending solely to the bodily 'nature' of man. If a moral theology based on such a limited understanding of man were to engage in dialogue with the medical profession, then both physicians and theologians would be reading God's will simply from the *rôle* of biological processes. This is precisely what a great number of theologians and other churchmen read into article 10 of the encyclical *Humanae Vitae:* 'In relation to biological processes, responsible parenthood means the knowledge and the respect of their functions; the human intellect discovers in the power of giving life biological laws which are part of human nature.'

I think that it is possible to give this text an acceptable interpretation in the sense that biological processes must not be ignored, which medicine never does. Since they are a part of human nature, they must be taken into consideration, not as the final word, but as one aspect of man's life. However, footnote 9 to this text suggests the rather divergent view of the conservatives; it indicates that at least the drafters of the encyclical, or those who provided it with footnotes, believed that the biological processes by themselves manifest God's absolutely binding will. The footnote refers us to the *Summa Theologica* where it is said, among other things: 'omnia illa, ad quae homo habet naturalem inclinationem ratio naturaliter apprehendit ut bona, et per consequens ut opere consequenda. . . . Inest homini inclinatio ad aliqua magis specialia secundum naturam, in qua communicat cum ceteris animalibus: et secundum hoc dicuntur esse de lege naturali, quae natura omnia animalia docuit; ut est commixtio maris et feminae, et educatio liberorum, et similia'.

—'By nature, reason directs all towards man's natural inclinations and sees them as a good and consequently as an imperative goal of his action. . . . According to nature, man has an inborn inclination to some particular goods which he shares with all the other animals; and in this respect, there belongs to the natural law whatever nature teaches all the animals, for instance, the copulation of male and female and the rearing of children, and similar things'.[3]

For modern people, it is hardly conceivable that we can read from the common nature of animals the norm for marital intercourse and the rearing of children! That nature which man has in common with animals is the subject of biology and zoology but in no way does it specify an ethical norm. As for theology, it has no place in biology or zoology; its *rôle* is defined in the context of man's relationship to God and his fellowmen. What pertains only to the biological or zoological domain remains theologically neutral. Whenever the biological enters the human context, it also enters theology, and precisely at the point of a person's responsibility to God and to his fellowmen, that is, at the point specifically related to his vocational responsibility — in this case, the marital and parental vocation. The example of St Thomas Aquinas explaining the norms for sexuality on the basis of the unspecified nature of all animals points to the fact that ancient cultures had not yet come to grips with the specific character of human sexuality. It is noteworthy that the medicine of the thirteenth century had also a merely somatic view of illness.

If modern medicine has great admiration for the marvels of the biochemical world, it is truly astounded by the psychosomatic correlations of man's ailments. More than ever medicine is faced with the necessity of correcting biochemical processes and psychosomatic determinisms. This holds at the individual level and also in the social sector of prophylactic medicine. It is true that many corrections follow the indications of biological 'norms,' particularly in matters of merely somatic dysfunction or

---

[3] *Summa Theologica,* 1-2:94:2:e.

illness. These are actually the simplest cases in medical ethics and pose no specific moral problems.

The biological nature of man as a partial aspect of his being does not bear any definite normative character. It can never set an intangible limit but it does, very often, have an indicative character. In most situations, biological laws would stand the test of serving the good of the total person. Medicine usually imitates them or brings them to full function whenever possible, but it cannot always attain this goal. It is at this juncture that bold challenges and new questions confront modern medicine.[4]

Not only the natural-science school of medicine but particularly the anthropological school founded by great physicians and Christians opposes any kind of 'sacralization' of the physiological aspect of man's nature. Typical human health is the norm to which anthropological physicians are dedicated. The question, therefore, of the readability of God's will in human nature leads of necessity to another question: what is the best possible human health in view of man's total vocation? (this point will be treated at length in the last chapter). The best of modern medicine refuses any kind of absolutizing in relation to the somatic aspects of health if this is to the detriment of man's overall well-being and human dignity.

What can philosophy say in answer to our question? It points above all to the 'natura rationalis,' and for modern thinkers this means the sharing of experiences, continuous research and co-reflection. Man's nature must express and reflect developing experimentation and systematic attention to experience. In many things, the already accumulated experience and reflections of mankind give us a satisfactory or even a definite response, but many questions call for new experiences, experimentation and a rethinking.

Experimentation belongs more and more visibly to the very nature of man, and this is particularly true with respect to

---

[4] R. Kautzky, 'Der Arzt und der menschliche Leib,' *Azrt und Christ*, 13 (1967), 146.

medicine in either treatment or prophylaxis. Historicity, that is, being by becoming and becoming by being in the great stream of human history, does indicate a direction of meaning and of values. However, not all that man has today and not even all that constitutes his direction is already written in his existence as we now find it. Not everything has to be determined once and forever.

No concept of human nature is adequate without special attention to planning and foresight in view of man's great goals, of time-bound opportunities and attendant dangers. The importance of man's awareness in relation to his true vocation needs to be emphasized. The man of today realizes how evolution and the whole of contemporary society are moulding him in his biological structures and processes, and even more in his cultural capacities. The influence of culture and the geographical-environmental conditions of life do not always contribute to the well-being and total vocation of man. Humanity, therefore, appeals to responsible men in all fields of endeavour and particularly to physicians for appropriate corrective measures. A *laissez-faire* attitude towards evolving nature could constitute one of the most unforgivable sins.

Reference has already been made to theology's indefatigable efforts to understand the complexity of man's nature, his total vocation in the actual historical situation, in the reality of man who has a history, is history and must shape history. While seeking to read God's will for man in his pilgrim situation, we should heed the following points.

(1) If we speak of 'nature' as indicative or normative for morality, we must always be mindful of man's total nature, meaning and vocation. Emphasis on one aspect alone can never provide a definitive explanation.

(2) We need to be aware of the tremendous desacralizing powers of revelation and of the particular contribution of modern medicine in the destruction of taboos which prevented man from assuming full responsibility for his heritage and for the future of mankind. This desacralization that has freed man from age-

old taboos is countered by a great re-sacralization, that is, by the emphasis on the dignity of the human person, and on his identity and responsibility before God and his fellowmen. We assert the absolute sacredness or sanctity of man's capacity to reciprocate genuine love and to discern its implications and demands. We believe in the inviolability of man's religious nature expressed in his capacity to search for God, to love and adore him. We insist on the need of an incarnate approach to man's freedom and sense of duty. Responsibility for the world in which men are destined to live together is one of the most sacrosanct duties of man, infinitely more sacred than biological processes.

(3) Theology has become more aware that the historicity of man is a serious matter. Personal responsibility has to be seen in the light of the history of salvation which must never be cut off from the total history of the world and of mankind.

(4) Contemporary theology is aware of a legitimate pluralism in hierarchies of value based on the variety of historical cultures; there is even diversity in approach to the most sublime mysteries. Through historical studies we come to see that in whatever past theologies had to say about human nature as expressive of God's will, there are abiding elements which must be distinguished from the particular cultural aspects subject to change. An over-simplified discourse on 'How to read God's will from the given nature' could lead to the most abominable typing of a specific culture, a cultural colonialism detrimental to mankind.

D. *Medical manipulation: the search for valid criteria*

The conclusion is that no single aspect of man's life and meaning can be isolated from a perspective of wholeness if it is intended to lead to a valid discernment of the will of God for man. How does this insight apply to the much discussed problem of medical manipulation?

The concept of 'manipulation' is not as yet clearly defined. There is some agreement, however, on how to differentiate 'manipulation' from the more generic concept of medical 'intervention.' An interruption of pregancy or an amputation are interventions with the gravest of consequences but they are not called manipulations. That a number of interventions may be or are called manipulations is clearly contingent on the concept of human nature, and consequently, on the understanding of medical service. A classical medical intervention in view of the treatment of a bodily illness is not called manipulation. Psychoanalysis or psychotherapy intended to correct a pathological disturbance of psychogenic origin is not, in itself, a manipulation, but if it brings about a substantial change in the patient's character and psychological reactions in a direction opposed to wholesome personality integration, we regard it as manipulation in a pejorative sense.

Social psychology often refers to 'manipulation' in relation to advertising and public opinion. We distinguish responsible participation in the moulding of public opinion carrying with it a respect for the individuals involved from the tricky and dishonest methods of imposing on a populace one's own ideology or goals with no respect for its freedom and co-responsibility. This distinction may help towards a better understanding of the limits separating justified from unjustified medical manipulations.

In medical usage, the word 'manipulation' is often used pejoratively. Whoever views biological processes as absolute ethical norms, condemns *ipso facto* all interventions modifying those processes as manipulations. For others the same measure of interference can be judged affirmatively and the word 'manipulation' may even take on a favourable connotation. It is often used to refer to a systematic attempt by man to modify, shape or reshape his genes, his biological heritage or his psychological reactions. So manipulation means more than a justified interference in view of therapy. It may refer in one case to an aggressive and somewhat irresponsible shaping or reshaping of man, and in another, to a beneficial shaping of the given 'material' of man's biological self or his psychic determinisms.

Effective means of birth regulation by chemical and mechanical devices are often labelled manipulation, since they go beyond therapy to pattern the whole fertility system. Ecclesiastical vocabulary refrains from using the term 'manipulation' if the reproductive system is conditioned by the calculated use of cyclical methods, although the same purpose is served. Outside ecclesiastical circles, however, this calculated control is properly called manipulation with all the possible connotations. Both sides state their arguments. The main reason advanced by churchmen is that the rhythm method does not intercept biological processes but consists only in a planned modification of the fecundity system along the lines of organic functions. In article 14 of their declaration in relation to the encyclical *Humanae Vitae,* the German bishops distinguished between the 'piloting' of the processes of life and those forms of 'manipulation' of life and sexual relationships that run counter to the dignity of the human person. I follow here those who carefully distinguish the two possible meanings of 'manipulation' as (a) a wise piloting, and (b) an arbitrary, unwise experimentation, attended by incalculable dangers of weakening man's heritage.

Would a perfect normalization of a woman's cycle by hypnosis, to the point of accurately determining the moment of ovulation, be considered a 'manipulation' or not? If chemical means could determine beyond all earlier expectations the accurate moment of ovulation, would their use be considered manipulation? These questions are posed as a warning against hair-splitting distinctions which could well jeopardize our credibility.

The discussion about the meaning, goal and limits of manipulation arose mainly from the fact that man is gaining greater power over his physiological, biological and psychosomatic 'nature.' Although the debate more often than not centres on organ transplantation, birth control and the new prospects of eugenic-genetic engineering, it is also extended into other fields, for instance, into that of psychoanalysis. The decisive point lies not in the vocabulary but in the appropriate criteria for discernment. Often, however, the vocabulary already reflects a given position or even a given *Weltanschauung.* What I have said earlier about the normative value and understanding of human nature points to the following:

1. In view of the undeniable fact that innumerable events and influences of the environment, particularly the by-products of technology and culture, are constantly shaping and changing the biosomatic and psychosomatic nature of man, and often not to his benefit, I cannot see why it should be immoral for man to intervene consciously with planning and corrective foresight. The image of God as revealed in the Old and the New Testaments does not allow us to accuse man of pride and rebellion if he is constantly searching and seeking to decode the secrets of nature, to apply all his knowledge and art to serve his own development and human vocation.

The physician of today no longer defines his *rôle* by the Hippocratic notion of 'servant of nature' or servant of the ordered potentialities and powers of nature. He is acquiring a greater consciousness of his own creative status. He increasingly considers himself an architect and sculptor of the given stuff of nature. He scrutinizes nature in its manifold trends of development, in its positive potentialities and dangers of decay, and he tries to meet all these by creative interventions. My first thesis, then, is that we should prefer a conscious and responsible moulding of the *physis* to all those changes that happen through lethargy or sloth. In more sociological terms, I favour 'planned' change over 'natural' change.

2. A realistic appraisal of information on scientific progress and responsibility obliges us to sound a warning against unlimited eugenic engineering and utopian dreams such as the euthenic utopia of breeding selectively particular types of men through the choice of sperm or ovule donors without any respect for man's vocation to marriage and family life. There are bounds set by limited knowledge and techniques, and others arising from man's dignity. Man must use his creative capacities only in dependence on God, that is, in a spirit of responsibility for history and for his vocation as a person in community. Man's increasing power over his own nature becomes an appeal to greater responsibility and to more thorough reflection on the meaning of human existence. I oppose myself radically to the utopia of the apostles of molecular biology who would like to

breed a new kind of automaton of the Huxleyan *Brave New World* type, or a man with a physical makeup that would enable him to live on other planets with total disregard for his humanity.

3. The main criterion is the principle of totality — not a totality of mere organic functions but a perspective of wholeness that considers the total vocation of the human person. It is not just a question of the meaning of the bodily organism; the most urgent issue relates to the meaning of an integral human life in response to man's earthly and eternal vocation.

In the past, medical ethics used the principle of totality to a great extent but only in view of a somatic concept of health and somatic medicine. If some drastic interventions sought solely the restoration of the impaired organ, they were inevitably justified by their utility to support or to correct defective nature, *cf.* Pope Pius XII in his discourse on progesterone treatment (September 12, 1958). After his pronouncement, moral casuistry sanctioned hormone therapy for the normalization of the biological cycle or for guaranteeing that ovarian rest or repose which in other circumstances would obtain 'naturally' through regular breast-feeding. Thus, either the justification of a chemical intervention failed to consider first the well-being of the mother, or else it disregarded it completely; moral casuistry was content to canonize physiological processes.

The traditional use of the principle of totality justified intervention in view of physical health and functioning. Medical ethics for the future must rest on an all-embracing concept of 'totality': *the dignity and well-being of man as a person in all his essential relationships to God, to his fellowmen and to the world around him.* In view of the breadth and depth of the human vocation, man can and must use his knowledge and art to manipulate the chaotic forces of the *physis* for the creation of a more humane order not only in the physical world but also in his psychosomatic nature. If it is more humane, it is also more pleasing to God. The mere observance of the impersonal and sub-personal laws and tendencies of 'nature' cannot guarantee such an increasingly humane order of development.[5]

God has entrusted to man his nature and his psychosomatic ordering for gradual submission to himself in the pursuit of his highest aspirations and for meeting the exigencies of his total vocation. Man must gradually emerge and remain above them. Instead of passively accepting natural determinisms in all their imperfections, he is to transform them as the materials of responsible stewardship, shaping and reshaping them in the service of his integral vocation.[6] Human culture involves not only man's ingenious interventions in the use of things, but also the planning of his own psychosomatic being. Culture depends very much on how man shapes himself in his longing and striving for a higher and higher degree of human development.

In the moulding of individuals and of culture, and especially in the problem of medical manipulation, we constantly have to view man in his wholeness, including the fullness of his vocation. The *whole* that is decisive as criterion is not the body, because it does not exist by itself. We deal either with a whole man or with a corpse. Neither is wholeness something outside the person — the nation, the society or the economic system — but the whole man himself in his individual and social existence, in his bodily, psychological and spiritual dimensions, in his capacity to build up a community of persons in love and justice, and to mould the world around him to the benefit of all human beings.

Each intervention or medical provision that helps or enhances the wholeness of the human person is right — be it a plastic heart or any other fantastic feat.[7] If, for instance, genetic engineering can eliminate the XYY chromosomal anomaly and thus protect humanity from the heavy burden of dangerous criminal tendencies in a number of people, why should we object

[5] Hans Rotter, S.J., 'Die Manipulation des Menschen,' *Arzt und Christ*, 16 (1970), 28.

[6] H. Thielicke, 'Ethische Fragen der modernen Medizin,' *Langenbecks Archive für klinische Chirurgie*, 321 (1968), 6.

[7] R. Kautzky, 'Der Arzt...' *op. cit.*, *Arzt und Christ*, 13 (1967), 145.

F

to it? If we can go a step further and imagine that the introduction of a new element into the chromosomes would give man greater stability or psychological balance or an increased power to bear suffering, would this constitute unjust manipulation? I do not think so.

If I say that the decisive norm or criterion is the human person and not the nation or society, it is because I categorically exclude the concept of mere efficiency, utility, and all kinds of manipulation that would sacrifice the person to an ideology or to a goal militating against man's dignity and true vocation. I want also to exclude a misconception or misunderstanding of man which would smack of individualism. Reference is to the whole man, the person in his highest capacity to reciprocate genuine love and to exercise responsibility. What I intend is the human person in the process of self-actualization through encounter with and in dedication to other persons, man engaged in shaping the world about him and in adoration of God. Manipulation would go beyond proper limits were it to cause man to deteriorate in these essential relationships. Medicine is always bound to respect the identity and authenticity of the person.

Chapter 6

THE LIFE OF MAN

The familiar yet mystifying phenomena of life and death have obsessed men from time immemorial. What is their meaning? Does bodily life *per se* have any significance? How is life entrusted to the patient and his physician? Is life the highest of all values? What guarantees its ultimate value?

By vocation, the physician is led to a co-reflection with his patient who is confronted by these questions in times of illness. He offers whatever assistance he can with the characteristic confidence and ethos of a man dedicated to the protection of life because of his respect and deep concern for it. The physician cannot, however, fulfil this great humane mission without realizing how each patient assesses his life as he faces illness and the prospect of death.

In his medical practice, the physician accumulates considerable experience in relation to the highly varied attitudes of people towards existence. Like the priest, the doctor soon comes to realize that life and death do not mean the same to everyone. While the last moments of some persons manifest an astonishing maturity, trust in God and unselfish interest in others as they utter a final wholehearted 'yes' to the Lord's calling in death,

others who did not value life equally are found totally unprepared
or unwilling to plumb the meaning of their imminent death.

The present discussion of life will examine and probe the
depths of its meaning for every man and particularly from the
point of view of medical ethics.

A. *The meaning of bodily life*

Bodily life is an exalted good. Before all material and
external goods, man's prime concern is for his own life. The
Christian considers the period of his earthly pilgrimage as the
unique *kairos,* that is, the time of favour, in which he is tried
and tested, the time allotted for growth in the love of God and
of his neighbour, the opportunity to transmit everlasting values
to many of his fellows and to give the best of himself for the benefit of mankind today and of future generations. It is the time to
incarnate values in his own being as well as in human history,
to personify love, goodness, joy, peace, justice and so on.
Eternally, man will be what he has made of himself during his
bodily life; the new heaven and the new earth will bear the
marks of the love he has embodied during his earthly mission.

The believer cannot consider his terrestrial journey in a
purely individualistic perspective as if it were merely the occasion
for him to save his soul and to prepare for an other-worldly
reward. Confronting life in its transcendent dimensions, he
realizes the uniqueness of the call to deploy his talents in the
Lord's world and to labour in his vineyard as a member of the
redeemed human family. This he accomplishes within a certain
culture as a bearer of the greatness and the misery of past history
and as a co-creator of the future of many.

Each day of life is precious. 'While daylight lasts we must
carry on the work' (Jn 9:4). In union with Christ whom
the Father willed should reveal through his earthly life the sense of
our own, and in the light of the Word Incarnate, the Redeemer
of the world, we come to understand more and more clearly the
momentous value of this short period of bodily life. For the

believer, it represents a gift and a constant appeal to 'make the most of the time' (Eph 5:16). It provides time either to prepare for an everlasting harvest in the community of the saints or for final dissolution in the solidarity of sin. 'For we must all have our lives laid open before the tribunal of Christ, where each must receive what is due to him for his conduct in the body, good or bad' (II Cor 5:10).

Our bodily life does not belong to us but to the One who has entrusted it to us for ourselves and for the service of our brethren. 'For no one of us lives, and equally no one of us dies, for himself alone. If we live, we live for the Lord; and if we die, we die for the Lord' (Rom 14: 7-8). Life, then, means existence in the saving solidarity of Christ with all men. Our life is entirely in God's hands — he can summon us at any moment. An awareness of our radical contingency strengthens the urgent appeal to use present opportunities. Readiness for God's final call is expressed by man's appreciation of each instant of his lifetime, and by vigilance for each favoured moment, in order to give our life its fullest sense in the service of others.

The Old Testament looks upon a long life as a gift of God, a blessing often inherent in the right use of this earthly life. 'Honour your father and your mother, that you may live long in the land' (Ex 20:12; Eph 6: 2-3). 'I will satisfy him with length of days' (Ps 91:16). 'The fear of the Lord brings length of days; the years of the wicked are few' (Prov 10:27). However, in the final analysis, the blessing of life consists not so much in longevity on earth as the good use of one's lifetime. They are graced who lived a fulfilled though short life (Wis 4:13). Man often bemoans the frailty of his earthly existence when it seems to fall short of attaining its plenitude; he is unable to decipher the riddle and asks God why 'in the prime of my life I must pass away; for the rest of my years I am consigned to the gates of Sheol' (Is 38:10). A full response lies not in God's graciously adding some years, but in Christ's commending his youthful life into the hands of the Father. By doing so in the greatest freedom, he gives to his life and to that of his followers the most sublime meaning: 'There is no greater love than this, that a man lay down his life for his friends' (Jn 15: 13).

The Gospel is explicit in stating that physical life is not the supreme good; it attains its truth and authenticity to the extent that it serves our neighbour and thus praises God, the giver of life. Our earthly mission is a call to eternal life, a summons to union with God here on earth and in the here-after, unity with God who is at once life and love. The man who is concerned solely with preserving his physical life loses his true self; the meaning of life eludes him as he disengages himself from sharing in God's life-giving love (Mt 8: 35; Lk 9: 34 and 17: 32; Jn 12: 25).

In a culture where kinship and bodily life supersede all other values, the warning of the Lord is harshly phrased: 'If anyone comes to me and does not hate his father and mother, wife and children, brothers and sisters, even his own life, he cannot be a disciple of mine' (Lk 14: 26). Of course, we are not to spurn blood relationships as such, nor life as a gift of God, but that tendency is worthy of contempt which renders absolute one's earthly life or mere blood solidarity to the detriment of a proper scale of values, particularly of personal freedom. During his terrestrial life, man's body and spirit come to everlasting fullness by unselfish devotion and occasionally even by sacrificial love. Christ reveals himself as the bearer of life by laying down his bodily life as a good shepherd (Jn 10: 11). Therefrom springs the believer's conviction that the greatest fulfilment of his earthly pilgrimage lies in his becoming more and more fully a sharer of the divine life by dedicating himself in love for the life of the world.

By making *life*, as such, the key concept of its saving message, the New Testament excludes any fragmentation, any one-sided consideration of the vegetative, biochemical or even psychosomatic dimension of earthly bodily life. These aspects are not to be neglected since their full meaning derives from an integral vision of the total human vocation. In the fullness of life as a central integrative reality each dimension falls into its proper place in the hierarchy of values.

B. *Man's stewardship of his life*

Man's bodily life is entrusted to his freedom as its most precious talent. He is not the independent lord of his life but only a steward subject to the sovereignty of God. Christ typifies the extent to which man can dispose of his life: he can even lay it down, if need be, in the service of his fellowmen as a witness to faith, hope and love. In placing his earthly life at the service of brotherhood, man gives the most authentic testimony that he appreciates life as a gift of God. He embraces unselfish devotion as the pivotal expression of that love which unites him to God, the origin and goal of his life.

Earthly life lies constantly exposed to manifold dangers. Those who yield to excessive concern about bodily risks weaken themselves through hypochondria and neurotic insecurity complexes. The mother who constantly watches over her children to ward off all possible risks deprives them of vitality and joy in life. Human life is altogether impossible without a free risk of bodily loss in the quest for life's meaning. The decisive question becomes: when may man risk his life and to what extent can the risk be justified?

So it is a matter of weighing values or ideals, and a question of prudence in discerning the right proportion between risk and anticipated result. The risks of mountain climbing, auto-racing and boxing are generally approved in our contemporary culture, but they are not to be judged on the same basis as the risk of doctors or nurses who expose their life and health in the course of their professional ministrations. Nor is the risk in sports comparable to self-experimentation by doctors; the latter contributes enormously to medical progress for the benefit of countless men.

The most carefully planned trip to the moon involving tremendous expenditures of talent and money may involve no more risk than auto-racing. The basic question remains always: is the expected benefit to mankind proportionate to the risk? The greater the love with which man risks his life, and the higher the service rendered for the common good or for a particular fellowman, the purer is the witness to faith and hope, and the more justifiable the risk. A relatively high degree of risk is praiseworthy when it is a matter of saving another's life.

Suicide strikingly contradicts the *rôle* of man as the faithful steward of his life. If, however, we pronounce such a harsh judgment on suicide, it is because of the decisiveness of such a drastic end, and the word 'suicide' can vary in significance according to the whole context and intent of the person who deprives himself of earthly life. In Dostoievsky's novel, *The Demons*, the suicide seeks the strongest proof available for expressing his rejection of God and asserting that he is the supreme master. He alone can dispose of his life, and thus, supposedly, assumes a divine attribute — though self-destruction is indeed a strange attribute to ascribe to God.

Suicide does not usually arise from such reflections but is an act of despair. The suicide is often a person who has failed to find the meaning of his life, or realizes that, at the moment in question, he has muddled it and made it senseless through a whole series of frivolous decisions and complications. A short-circuit has plunged his life into total darkness from which he fails to emerge. At the decisive moment, the basic instinct of self-preservation yields to tremendous frustration.

One who consciously and freely destroys his life is nothing other than a craven deserter who refuses to face the trials of the pilgrim. We must be mindful, however, that in spite of the extreme gravity of the sin of suicide, taken objectively, we may not and cannot judge the subjective guilt of anyone who has wrought self-destruction or attempted to do so. In many cases there is an acute mental disturbance. In fact, in justice and charity, we always assume this to be the case where those whom we know to have led a virtuous life have committed suicide in a moment of deep depression or under terrible compulsion.

The refusal of ecclesiastical burial which was so common in the past may have served as a useful deterrent, but in the light of today's psychology, we must regret the added anguish that this sanction often brought to the families concerned, while it is likely that it led to a thoroughly unjust moral judgment. Today, no priest will refuse ecclesiastical burial to a person who participated in the life of the Church should there be any indication that he acted in a moment of overwhelming depression. Doctors fulfil a duty of justice and charity towards the family by giving testimony to this probability.

In many cases of suicide the blame might well be laid at the door of society or of a particular environment, for despair often reflects the failure of those who should have shown justice and tender care for the despairing person. One need only think of so many old people living an isolated existence as if rejected by their families and by society, or of war veterans who do not receive enough assistance to lead a dignified and satisfying human life. Humanity in many corners of the world has lost strength and shows a weakened power to bear suffering. The community at large has lost its understanding and appreciation of the meaning of suffering.

A man faced with the case of a suicidal neighbour can well ask himself if, in conscience, he has a right or duty *to save the life of his neighbour* even against the latter's will. The answer, not only of the Christian but of the whole humanist tradition, is that there is such a duty, one of the reasons being the high probability that the person contemplating suicide is unable at that moment to make a truly personal decision. However, the help which the doctor or any friend may offer cannot be restricted to saving the biological life; rather, all efforts should be directed towards helping the prospective suicide to find the sense of his life and then arrive at a responsible decision.

Persons who suffer from compulsive suicidal tendencies or who fear that they may yield to their self-destructive impulse can often be helped by a 'significant other' who, by appealing to the best in them, brings into relief their positive qualities. Although we refrain from judging that an act under such compulsion would endanger their eternal life, they should be helped in building their self-confidence to the point where they can successfully overcome their compulsions and come to the fulfilment of their earthly vocation. The very fact that we do our best to save their life conveys a message to them that we still value them as persons.

The doctor who attends an attempted suicide wishes to give him a new chance for a fulfilled life, be it only through an act of sorrow and trust in God's mercy. Therefore, the physician will muster all his knowledge and art to bring the patient to that degree of serenity and capacity for free decision without which his life cannot attain its goal.

We should be most cautious in pronouncing the shocking word 'suicide'. Not only should we be aware of the legitimate limits of reductionism but also of the easily wounded sensitivity of relatives and friends. Faced with such a tragedy, we have to avoid any language that would seem to pass judgment. While today we understand that most suicides are triggered by unbearable mental distress, we should go beyond that, and appreciate, better than did the moralists of the past, that taking one's life can have all shades of meaning from throwing away one's 'worthless' life to giving one's life for a greater cause.

Socrates who, unjustly condemned, took the deadly drink according to the law of his country, became his own executioner, but he was not a suicide. The Japanese pilots who assured the success of their attacks on ships and other military targets by plunging themselves and their aircraft onto their objectives could not but lose their lives. Their direct intention, however, was not self-destruction but a noble military gesture that demanded self-sacrifice.

Between the two extremes of giving one's precious life in the service of love and casting away a life deemed futile, there are many nuances which should not be neglected and which cannot be encompassed by the one term 'suicide'. Even among the limited cases which one physician encounters in his practice, there is a tremendous difference in the suicidal patients' background, motives, ailments, disturbances, and so on.

There are many situations where a patient, by refusing to submit to a life-saving procedure, poses to the physician a

dilemma analogous to that posed by a prospective suicide. Is
the doctor duty-bound to act against the expressed unwillingness
of the person and save that life? The common conviction of
physicians is that not only has he the right but also the duty to
proceed with the life-saving operation when it is not extraordinary, all too expensive or too risky a process. The reasoning is
quite similar to that in the case of attempted suicide in that the
patient refusing a normal life-saving intervention is incompetent,
devoid of insight or even psychologically incapable of decision.
Only if, in a moment of full consciousness and deliberation, a
patient has expressed his will to accept death now rather than
the somewhat dubious prolongation of his life must his decision
be respected.

It is interesting to consider the newness of many aspects of
this question. In earlier times when painless and aseptic procedures were not possible, there was far less probability of saving
a patient's life. Almost invariably, brachial force had to be used
to immobilize the patient during the dreadful and painful
surgical procedures. Today, life-saving and pain-relieving interventions have become normal procedure. However, in view of
the fact that in many cases men have a lowered capacity for
enduring pain, it is understandable that their desire to live is
greatly reduced.[1] The physician's decision will be based on the
prospect of the patient's finding meaning in his life and sufficient
courage to assume its burden.

C. *Life entrusted to the love and justice of others*

From man's social nature it follows that accountability for
life is indubitatively a shared responsibility. Central to this truth
is the total dependence of the embryo, the fetus, the infant and
the little child on the acceptance and care of the mother. The
most reprehensible violation of co-responsibility in this respect

---

[1] M. Kohlhaas, 'Lebensrettung wider Willen?,' *Münchener Medizinische Wochenschrift*, 42 (1967), 2176-2179.

is infanticide, the killing by the mother or others of a child already born. However, a certain type of infanticide committed by the mother shortly after parturition can be explained by modern psychology as a psychopathological reaction. In most of these cases, the responsibility or culpability of the mother is sharply reduced if not nil. Often the environment shares the guilt for having made it psychologically so difficult for the mother to accept the impending *rôle* of parent and/or the child itself.

Historically, infanticide has played a horrifying *rôle*. Very often, a male-centred society would accept only a limited number of female children. In other societies, weak and crippled children were abandoned and left to die of exposure. That the social problem of infanticide came to be practically eradicated is due in no small measure to the Christian religion with its redeeming message for all human persons.

In today's world, medical competence saves the life of innumerable babies who are deformed, or abnormal in other ways: babies who, in other epochs, would unavoidably have died in spite of all the good will of their parents to accept them. Admirable efforts and a great expenditure of skill, time and money are invested here, at times perhaps more than warranted, because they are out of proportion to the subsequent efforts and expense necessary to help seriously-maimed children attain social adjustment and relatively normal personality development.

In spite of such disproportion, we cannot conclude that infants with a poor eugenic heritage or those afflicted by marked deformity should be condemned to death. Who would want to pass a death sentence on them? Only through faith in the dignity of each person will the medical profession and mature parents find the golden mean. On the one hand, no man has a right to declare another human life meaningless, worthless, and therefore condemned to death, since man's dignity does not depend on his efficiency or his capacity to contribute to the economy. On the other hand, when the 'life' of extremely disabled and abnormal children means practically no more than a vegetative existence, they need not, and sometimes should not, be sustained in life by all means available to modern medicine.[2]

The medical profession in today's world encompasses the task and vocation of saving lives threatened by social negligence, ineptitude or injustice, as in traffic and industrial casualties, individual and mob violence, dire poverty and the like. The pain endured by physicians faced in their daily experience by innumerable tragedies which could have been avoided by stricter and better-enforced laws and a better-informed public opinion oblige them to assume leadership in warning a society which could and should manifest greater respect for life by taking the necessary measures to protect it.

D. *The beginning of human life*

If the genesis of life has always fascinated man, speculation about the beginning of *human* life has consistently exceeded all other because of the interest of parents who are cooperators in the transmission of life and who care for existing life. The concern of physicians comes from their special vocation as 'servants of human life,' and the fact that throughout history, they have earnestly sought to know more about the inception of life. Moralists on their part have generally tended to adopt the opinions and convictions of physicians about the moment at which human life begins.

During the past centuries many circumstances favoured a growing conviction among Catholics that the 'ensoulment' of the embryo occurred at the moment of fertilization, that is, that life began at that instant. Conception as a privileged moment is celebrated as the beginning of Christ's human life (the Annunciation, March 25) and that of his mother (the Immaculate Conception, December 8). However, the moment of 'ensoulment' of a blastocyst or embryo does not belong to the data of revela-

---

[2] Bernard Häring, 'Hoffnungslose Krankheit und christliche Hoffnung,' *Die gegenwärtige Heilsstunde* (Freiburg, 1964), pp. 414-422.

tion or to any dogma. A certain awareness of this fact is discernible in the *Pastoral Constitution on the Church in the Modern World:* 'Therefore from the moment of its conception life must be guarded with the greatest care, while abortion and infanticide are unspeakable crimes' (GS, Art 51). The text which had been prepared for the second to last vote read: 'Life in the womb of the mother (*in utero*). . . .' A number of Council fathers proposed amendments 'that the expression *in utero* be deleted since the fertilized egg which is not yet in the uterus is sacred.' Others asked that a clearer distinction of 'abortion' be made. The response of the commission was that the text should read: 'from the moment of its conception'; this explained the intention, 'without touching upon the moment of animation.'[3] The commission also felt that it could not easily fulfil the demand for an accurate technical definition of abortion,[4] since it is not within the compass of the magisterium of the Church to settle the question of the precise moment after which we are faced with a human being in the full sense. Here we rely on the data of science and on philosophical reflection.

Traditionally there are two different opinions. The theory of the embryo's 'successive ensoulment' first with a vegetative, then with an animal and finally with a human soul, was the more commonly accepted before St Albert the Great. He rejected it in favour of *instant* or *simultaneous animation,* which asserts that an immortal soul is given at the very moment of procreation. But St Thomas Aquinas and his school still held to the theory of successive animation. The majority of theologians have followed the biologists and physicians who, over the last centuries, have become more and more convinced that the human principle of life was given at the time or at the very moment of fertilization. It is only of late that there no longer exists a consensus among biologists and physicians.

Our discussion would be incomplete without a brief exposition of the different theories of the origin of human life in the

---

[3] *Expensio Modorum.* Partis secundae. Resp. 101, a and c, p. 36.
[4] *Ibid.*

light of modern embryology. The inception of new life highlights four decisive moments in the early developmental stages of man: (a) the origin of the genotype; (b) the time of possible segmentation in the case of identical twins; (c) the time of implantation and (d) the development of the typically human cerebral cortex. Later discernible signs of development of the fetus, such as its quickening and the hour of birth, are lesser disjunctions in the course of the transmission and unfolding of human life. The gross estimates of the old Mediterranean world about 'ensoulment' or hominization around the fortieth day for boys and eightieth day for girls are totally outdated.

1. *The origin of the genotype*

The first decisive moment of new life is the moment of fertilization of the ovum. At this moment, a new life, distinct from that of the father and that of the mother is given, with a unique, never-to-be-repeated genetic code. It is a minute, microscopic speck containing a multitude of inherited characteristics. A virtually infinite number of combinations of paternal and maternal traits are excluded in favour of those which will determine the individuality of the new life and the innate potentialities that can unfold during its earthly existence. The genotype has been determined.

The blastocyst then develops its own dynamics of life, separate from that of the mother. After five to seven days of cell division in the tube, the zygote finds its way to the uterus where it pursues its own activities and creates an environment compatible with further development. The most astonishing feature of this stage is the self-reproductive power of the cells, each marked by the same genotype and the most marvellous entelechy. The blastocyst itself simultaneously takes on the two great tasks of implantation and further embryonic development. The outline of the placental system and amniotic sac is already in the blastocyst. The ectodermal layer of one of its folds, called the trophoblast, burrows into the uterine lining and the zygote nestles there. This pole is to become the placenta, an essentially fetal system; the opposite pole becomes the embryo. So the blastocyst, by its fore-ordained cellular power, is throwing out a lifeline by which it will be attached to the bloodstream of the mother. Before its implantation, it already has its own communication network sending hormonal information into the maternal host-organism, thus inviting it to prepare for that forthcoming solidary life during nine months.

All this miraculous dynamism inclusive of the whole system of communication suggests the presence of the principle of life which is to unfold and to manifest itself eventually in the fully developed child and adult person. What characterizes the whole process is the tremendous surpassing of present forms into new ones of greater complexity and more astonishing unity. The principle of this transcendence is *inborn*, although its dynamic activity can unfold only in the appropriate environment and in constant communication with it. Thus, by now and on this level, there is a dialectical or 'dialogical' principle expressed at the stage of life which is embodied.

These data of embryology seem to buttress the position of biologists, philosophers and moralists who consider fertilization as the precise and most decisive moment in the transmission of human life. They are convinced that everything is directed by a typically human life principle which we may call 'soul' or the life-breath of the person.

2. The time of segmentation

The greatest objection to the theory of 'ensoulment' at the time of fertilization is posed by the phenomenon of identical twins. Segmentation, which is the great event of biparous gestation, occurs at about the same time as implantation. The problem lies in the fact that a personal life can be given only if there is complete individualization. Identical twins represent two individualities though with the same genotype. If all human offspring arose in pairs as identical twins, it would be logical enough to consider the moment of segmentation or final individualization as the most characteristic moment of incipient human life.

The process of segmentation that leads to twinning or multiple births can happen at different stages:

(a) The separation can happen at the morular stage, *i.e.*, at about the eighth cell division in the tube, or on the zygote's way out of the tube on the fourth or fifth day after fertilization. In this case, each twin or triplet will form its own placental system and burrow itself into the walls of the uterus at different places.

(b) Segmentation can happen immediately before, during, or immediately after implantation so that the twins have the same placental system. This is the more common occurrence with identical twins.

(c) In some rare cases, the division of the two or more embryos need not happen until the second half of the second week, *i.e.*, until the twelfth or fourteenth day after fecundation. Then the twins also share the same amniotic sac. In these unusual cases it can also happen that the division is incomplete or imperfect, so that the twins are joined in some portion of the body.

Recently, another phenomenon has been observed which casts further doubt on the thesis which asserts that the fertilized ovum has that degree of individualization without which a personal being is nonexistent. 'Twinning in the human being may occur up to the fourteenth day, when conjoined twins can still be produced. Less well known is the fact that in these first few days the twins or triplets may be recombined into one individual being.'[5] In the case of mice, this recombination of several fertilized eggs into one individual embryo can happen up to the thirty-second cell division stage. With human beings, it is not yet known how long (up to which mitotic stage) this is possible. 'All these matters are brought forth to point out that although at fertilization a new genetic package is brought into being, within the confines of one cell, this anatomical fact does not necessarily mean that all this genetic material becomes crucially

---

[5] A. E. Hellegers, 'Fetal Development,' *Theological Studies*, 31 (1970), 4

G

activated at that point or that irreversible individuality has been achieved.[6]

The consequence seems obvious: without individualization there is no personalization, that is, there has not yet emerged a human person. We must be careful however in drawing our conclusions about those blastocysts which actually do not engage in a process of twinning or recombination. Is it that they lack the potentiality for such a process, namely, a genetic code for twins? If so, there could be real individualization. Or is it a case of an adequate genetic code for twinning awaiting some form of activation? In the latter situation, we should be able to assert categorically that the process of individualization is not yet fully achieved. It needs to be stressed that only a human individual can have the quality of a person.

3. Implantation

Through implantation in the womb of the mother, the blastocyst obtains its natural habitat. It emerges from a rather striking insecurity and loneliness to the point of a life-saving attachment and acceptance by the maternal host. Actually, it is at this point that the woman becomes mother in the fullest sense, namely, through acceptance of the blastocyst into her own system. The estimates of qualified scientists are that thirty to fifty per cent of fertilized cells get lost before implantation, while the rate of loss from the time of implantation to birth is in the ten to twenty per cent probability range. Nature's prodigality in the early stages accounts for the fact that many scientists and philosophers do not believe personhood to be given with such a greatly diminished chance of ever coming to full development and conscious personal life.

Others argue in a more philosophical vein insisting on the dialogical or dialectical character of the human person: 'A person is more than being an individual cell. To-be-a-person means essentially *relationships* including human persons as well

---

[6] *Ibid.*, p. 5.

as the fundamental relationship of man to God (transcendence).
The human body is the foundation and symbol (Real-symbol)
of this transcendence to the other. The implantation makes this
self-transcendence transparent in a special way.' [7] One of the
conclusions drawn by proponents of this scientific position is that
in vitro experimentation with fertilized eggs would not be
ontogenesis of a human being but merely a breeding of proto-
plasmic material.[8]

While I can see the highly symbolic and real values of the
acceptance of the blastocyst by the mother's endometrium, I
feel that the argument based on it is an overstatement of the
case if it asserts that implantation is the definitive moment of
the ontogenesis of the human person. At least, as long as this
argument stands alone without further scientific corroboration
and insight, it remains unconvincing to me.

4. *The cerebral cortex and hominization*

The newer theories about 'brain death' as the termination of
human life bring into prominence another theory about the
beginning of life. This posits the development of the typically
human cerebral cortex as the decisive phenomenon in the ontogenesis of the human person. At this point, I depend for the
most part on the articles of Ruff [9] and the authoritative work of
Glees.[10]

Besides the high mortality rate of blastocysts and
embryos in the first weeks, there is above all the fact of the

---

[7] F. Böckle, 'Um den Beginn des Lebens,' *Arzt und Christ*, 14 (1968), 70.
   Böckle relies, for instance, on G. Sauser and M. Vodipivec, 'Mediko-
   theologische Anmerkungen zum Problem der Humanontogenese,' *Gott
   und Welt*. Festgabe für Karl Rahner. Vol. II (Freiburg, 1964),
   pp. 850-872.
[8] E. Chiavacci, 'Riflessioni per una morale della manipolazione
   dell'uomo,' *Rivista di teologia morale*, 8 (1970), 28.
[9] Wilfried Ruff, S.J., 'Individualität und Personalität im embryonalen
   Werden,' *Theologie und Philosophie*, 45 (1970), 24-59. 'Das em-
   bryonale Werden des Menschen,' *Stimmen der Zeit*, 181 (1968),
   331-355.
[10] P. Glees, *Das menschliche Hirn* (Stuttgart, 1968).

anencephalic fetus (one characterized by the lack of the essential parts of the brain), for which no personal activity whatsoever can be possible. Personal life manifests its nature or essence through consciousness, self-reflection, thought and free decision. Human consciousness has an indispensable substratum in the cerebral cortex. According to important paleontological and anthropological findings, the human species transcended itself by a tremendous leap in the development of the cerebral cortex which distinguishes man from all animals, and without which no manifestation of specifically human personal attributes or activity is conceivable.[11]

The decisive question is now: can a living being be a person at all without the development of the biological conditions and/or presuppositions of personal life? [12] The theory just discussed considers implantation as cause and symbol of the beginning of dialogical existence, but is this theory based on the marvellous unity between living body and life-breath or spiritual principle which we discussed in the preceding chapter? The soul is not pre-existent to the body; this is common conviction. Does it then come into existence as a mere spiritual principle without a corresponding body, as Hellenistic thinking would suggest? The question concerns the beginning of a human person existing in the body and through the body, and prepared to express itself only in and with the body, at least in this earthly life. But the cerebral cortex is now accepted as the central organ of all personal manifestations and activities.

Between the fifteenth and fortieth day, there develops the basic structure of a typically human cerebral cortex, although not fully unfolded. During this time, and particularly between the fifteenth and twenty-fifth day, there are still numerous developmental failures which normally lead to spontaneous rejection of the embryo by the mother-organism. It seems that in these cases the ontogenesis of the human person did not

---

[11] Teilhard de Chardin, 'The Birth of Thought,' *The Phenomenon of Man* (New York: Harper and Row, 1965), pp. 163-190.
[12] Ruff, *Theologie und Philosophie, op. cit.,* p. 43.

succeed. It is most unusual (one case in a thousand) for the organism of the mother to keep and nourish an anencephalic fetus.

A further aspect is not without interest. Today it is possible to preserve living cells of the human body and even to bring about continued mitotic division. There is evidently no personal life centre but there is a biological centre without which cells could not live and develop. These cell cultures contain the whole genetic code of a person but there is no individualization.

Further, if the human brain is deprived of oxygen for a maximum of ten minutes, the lower and more primitive part of the brain which sustains biological life processes can be reactivated through resuscitation procedures, but the loss of activity of the cortical centres is irreversible; there can be no further conscious life. Medical science then speaks of 'brain death.' The question then arises: does it not follow that before the formation of the typically human cerebral cortex there exists merely a biological centre of life bereft yet of the substratum of a personal principle?

The basic structure of the human cerebral cortex is *outlined* between the fifteenth and twenty-fifth (or at least after the fortieth) day of normal development. By eight weeks, there is detectable electrical brain activity. By twelve weeks, the brain structure is complete. Most probably we can conclude that after the twenty-fifth or at least after the fortieth day there is no qualitative leap but only a quantitative development of the already given structure of the cerebral cortex. Between the twenty-fifth to the fortieth day after fertilization and the first year of life, there is a marvellous maturation of the cerebral cortex but there is not that self-transcendence or leap in the basic brain structure that marks the third to fourth week of embryonic development or eventually the third to twelfth week of intra-uterine life. About one year after birth, the child has reached that quantitative development of the grey matter that allows him full self-consciousness and all the other characteristic spiritual qualities. Even a few days or weeks after birth, the infant smiles in a way which is phenomenally wonderful as an expression of the human person.

Repeatedly, this qualitative leap in the formation of the cerebral cortex has been compared with phylogenesis. It is not the same; radical differences exist. The ontogenesis of the embryo or fetus, *i.e.*, the development of the typically human cerebral cortex is no doubt a stupendous self-transcendence, an admirable leap, but each blastocyst encapsulates this innate tendency in spite of the fact that it is not always successful. Phylogenesis, on the contrary, is a quite extraordinary and unexpected leap prepared by a long history and willed, of course, by God. Supposing the validity of the theory 'that the spiritual soul comes into existence only in a later phase of embryonic development, this means that between fertilization of the ovum and the development of the organism with a spiritual life principle, there are certain biological phases which cannot yet be called man . . . then we might really say that such an ontogenesis does correspond to the human phylogenesis. In both cases, an organism that is not yet human is tending towards that complexification and condition in which the existence of the spiritual soul finds its biological substratum.' [13]

In view of all that has been explained about human life, that is, personal existence in a live body which is the substratum of the spiritual life principle, it does seem that the theory which presents hominization as dependent on the development of the cerebral cortex has its own probability. I think it can be said that at least before the twenty-fifth to fortieth day, the embryo cannot yet (with certainty) be considered as a human person; or, to put it differently, that about that time the embryo becomes a being with all the basic rights of a human person. At the present moment, however, this is no more than an opinion which deserves serious consideration and further discussion. If I may state my own opinion clearly on this point: the theory of hominization as dependent on the development of the cerebral cortex does not provide sufficient ground for depriving the embryo of the basic human right to life; but if this theory gains

---

[13] Karl Rahner and P. Overhage, *Das Problem der Hominisation* (Questiones disputatae 12/13). (Freiburg, 1961), p. 79.

general acceptance by those competent in the field, it could then contribute greatly to the resolution of those difficult cases involving conflict of conscience or conflict of duties.

E. Birth regulation as a medical problem

The value of human life and medicine's dedication and service to it have special relevance to questions concerning conception and contraception. Whereas we know from the history of medicine that the physician has always served couples desirous of fulfilling their parental vocation, the medical profession today views its service in terms not only of the restoration of biological fertility but also of its regulation. This compels the physician to situate his task in the broader context of the whole problematic of responsible parenthood in view of society and the future of humanity. The immediate concern of the physician however, is the health of persons who seek his assistance for the begetting of offspring in a responsible way.

I do not intend to treat here the whole problematic of birth regulation and the underlying concept of nature, since I have done this in other books.[14] I shall confine myself to the medico-ethical aspects of the problem in the light of medicine today.

1. Contraception is not abortion

In the eyes of alert representatives of modern medicine, the most unforgivable sin is failure to distinguish clearly between abortion and contraception as a means of birth regulation. Incredible as it seems, there is a trend among some physicians, and even more among leaders of planned parenthood organizations, to confuse these two totally different issues. That a poorly educated public also confounds them is less surprising.

---

[14] Bernard Häring, *Brennpunkt Ehe* (Bergen-Enkheim: Verlag Kaffke, 1968. *Love is the Answer* (Danville, N.J.: Dimension Books, 1970). *Paternità responsible* (Roma: Ed. Sales, 1970). *Married Love* (Chicago, Ill.: Argus Communications, 1969).

Although the sperm and the ovum are living cells, they lack all those qualities that characterize human life as human. The prospect of a possible parthenogenesis in no way weakens this statement; it would only focus our attention and knowledge on the moment of conception and would probably lead to greater accuracy in stating the moment of *conception* as the beginning of truly human life. A gamete differs qualitatively from a fertilized germinal cell with its dynamic process, and not merely quantitatively. This differential is true even when we pay full attention to the arguments of scientists who point to later qualitative leaps leading to the final individualization and to the development of the basic structure of the cerebral cortex. Our earlier discussion of the diverse theories bearing on the beginning of human life, in the sense of complete hominization, would not allow us to confuse contraception with interruption of pregnancy. If anything, it demands further distinction of the terms 'conception' and 'abortion'.

2. *Biological processes*

Medicine has great respect for biological facts, processes, trends and determinisms. If their functioning is defective or deficient, physicians try to restore it but only in so far as medical intervention serves the overall good of the person. It is an accepted rule of medicine not to interfere with biological processes or determinisms unless the well-being of the person demands it (cf. chapter 8). However, it would be contrary to the best standards of modern medicine to give higher priority to mere biological processes than to the psychological and psychosomatic. From the medical point of view, therefore, observance of the rhythm method which safeguards the biological processes better than most methods of birth control should be endorsed, and its practice should be facilitated eventually through further research. But wherever in a given culture and in concrete cases this method results in psychological damage to the general health and well-being of the person, a physician cannot reconcile its exclusive recommendation with total personal health and his service to it. This principle finds general applicability and is not restricted solely to cases of somatic disturbance of psychogenic origin. Whenever birth regulation seems to be mandatory in view of the patient's personal and family interests, the adverse psychological aftermath of a calculated periodical or enforced total continence *per se* will have to be comparatively evaluated with the probable biological and psychological effects of other methods.

3. *Therapy and birth regulation*

In view of the enormously complex situation of the birth control problem, it is a great blessing that Pope Paul did not give doctrinal sanction to a specific medical method. Otherwise, not only would he have overstepped the bounds of his competence but he would have had to shoulder responsibility for all the damage likely to ensue from that one method. It suffices to recall the court trial of the suppliers of thalidomide (contergan). Neither the Pope nor any episcopate wanted to assume responsibility for the indiscriminate use of progesterone pills. Whatever may be said about the questionable concept of natural law in the encyclical *Humanae Vitae*, the questions were properly approached under the heading of therapy. Medical methods are to be judged by medical competence and in terms of therapy, that is, of the probable results for the individual person and for the health of mankind.

It is incumbent on medical science to study all the effects of the rhythm method not only in reference to psychic equilibrium but also in view of any adverse consequences it may have for the offspring. Statistics advanced by physicians and scientists in the field of reproductive biology indicate that women who used the rhythm method exclusively had a higher percentage of defective children. A still unproved hypothesis relates the abnormality to 'over-aged' sperms and ova that have greatly decreased vitality; the incidence was tied in with intercourse on the limits of the 'safe' periods. Should this be the case, medical science has to advise a wider margin of security, possibly by prescribing periods of continence some days earlier. It is only one example of how each method has to be tested in a truly medical perspective. The mandate to do so comes from the scientific autonomy so strongly emphasized by the Second Vatican Council in its *Constitution on the Church in the Modern World* (GS, Art 36).

The statement of *Humanae Vitae* (Art 15) relative to the concept of therapy and the direct intention of putting an impediment to birth was the object of vehement discussion. The text reads: 'The Church, on the contrary, does not at all consider illicit the use of those therapeutic means truly necessary to treat diseases of the organism, even if an impediment to procreation which may be foreseen, should result therefrom, provided such impediment is not, for whatever motive, directly willed.' With respect to the direct intention to regulate birth, it has to be said that not only the conciliar document on *The Church in the Modern World* but also the Pope's encyclical stress the need for responsible transmission of life which, at times, means responsible avoidance of another pregnancy. Surely, contraception is to be excluded in cases where it would mean nothing other than condoning irresponsibility and selfishness. As to the method itself, the physician will judge according to the general concept of therapy, that is, in view of the best possible service to the person's health.

The English version 'truly necessary to treat diseases of the organism' (*corpus*) is to be explained according to the nature of man, the psychosomatic unity, the total concept of health and, consequently, according to therapy. The anthropological vision of medicine always embraces the overall well-being of the human person and chooses the method accordingly. In no way does this contradict the encyclical if we translate the Latin word 'corpus' in the sense which 'body' had in the Semitic tradition or has now in modern medicine. But equally, in the same perspective, medicine cannot ignore the results of a given method on the total development of the person, which includes, above all, moral development. Therefore, the physician cannot be indifferent to the norm of birth regulation given by the Council document, *The Church in the Modern World:* 'Therefore, when there is question of harmonizing conjugal love with the responsible transmission of life, the moral aspect of any procedure does not depend solely on sincere intentions or on an evaluation of motives. It must be determined by objective standards. These, based on the nature of the human person and his acts, preserve the full sense of mutual self-giving and human procreation in the context of true love' (GS, Art 51). The text refers to the nature of the person in his capacity to reciprocate genuine love and to fulfil the vocation of spouse or parent in a context that allows for growth in genuine love.

4. *Medical enlightenment*

A decision as important as birth regulation requires that the physician respect thoroughly the conviction and conscience of his patient. This does not exclude (on the contrary, it includes) imparting the information necessary from the point of view of medical competence and total health. Such a complex matter also demands that the physician be mindful of the limits of his professional and human competence. If in some aspects he is not fully informed, he will tell his patients so, admitting that he must seek further counsel from other competent colleagues. Beyond the medical aspect, cooperation among physician, marriage counsellor and priest is advisable. It would be an error on my part to give such advice to physicians only. It must be said emphatically to the priest or confessor that he has always to be conscious of his limited competence in the matter of health, especially in its psychosomatic and psychological ramifications and therapy.

Modern man will not easily tolerate or accept a physician's attempt to give a moralistic sermon to a patient seeking medical advice. By 'moralistic sermon' I understand an effort to impose abstract norms which, in his eyes, may be valid but which bear no relationship to his task as physician. Whenever, however, the physician finds that a naïve trust in artificial means for the resolution of all problems, an immature attitude, or a flight before conscience are causes of neurosis or psychosomatic disturbances, it rightly belongs to him to explain these interactions. Recourse to chemical-mechanical means or an astute calculation of the infecund periods without responsible attention to its effect on the marital relationship can be causes of neurotic impairment. It would not be 'moralizing' for a doctor to lead his patient to a fuller understanding of the whole human problem with all its moral implications.

5. *Sterilization*

Traditional moral theology has consistently distinguished between direct and indirect sterilization. Any sterilization with the stated intention of inducing a temporary or irreversible sterility was declared immoral, while sterilization necessary for healing organic ailments was declared licit. This approach, though sensible, is much too narrow. The vocabulary is hardly intelligible to medical thought today in view of the fact that the Church has given official sanction and encouragement to the principle of responsible parenthood, and has realized the tremendous relevance of marital relationships to the stability of a marriage and to the health and harmonious relationship of husband and wife. It might be said, then, that the real immorality comes in the irresponsible refusal to fulfil the vocation of husband and wife and of mother and father. The intention to carry out this base decision by sterilization must be absolutely rejected. But wherever the direct preoccupation is responsible care for the health of persons or for saving a marriage (which also affects the total health of all persons involved), sterilization can then receive its justification from valid medical reasons. If, therefore, a competent physician can determine, in full agreement with his patient, that in this particular situation a new pregnancy must be excluded now and forever because it would be thoroughly irresponsible, and if from a medical point of view sterilization is the best possible solution, it cannot be against the principles of medical ethics, nor is it against 'natural law' (*recta ratio*). The medical decision, however, cannot disregard the foreseeable or possible effects of vasectomy or tubal ligation upon the total health of the person subjected to this procedure.

If, for instance, the last two pregnancies of this woman have triggered a psychosis and there is no hope that her husband will act responsibly, tubal ligation may be the only or at least the best means of saving the mother for the fulfilment of her task as wife and mother in her already trying situation. There are many other cases of comparable gravity.

There are situations where the easier and more just solution would demand the sterilization of the husband, especially where moral judgment is based on evidence of impairment on his part and that, in conscience, he should not transmit life in the future; his wife, on the other hand, should he die, might responsibly desire a pregnancy in a later marriage. Of course, we cannot approve the sterilization of a husband for selfish reasons, for example, because he neither wants children nor accepts any form of self-control. Doctors are known to have told men who wanted to have their wives sterilized so as to avoid having a second or third child, 'why do you not get sterilized yourself since this is much easier for you and since you are the one who does not want children?' This seemed to be a very effective way to dissuade the inconsiderate husband. In other cases, a most thoughtful and responsible husband may choose to submit himself to the simpler operation when his wife's health or other grave reasons make it clear that to risk any more pregnancies would be irresponsible.

6. *Artificial insemination* [15]

In his 1949 address on medical ethics, Pius XII condemned artificial insemination in no uncertain terms.[16] The pope then found within the Catholic Church and beyond it widespread attention and agreement. If his condemnation is primarily directed against artificial insemination where the donor is not the husband, we have only to think of the abuse of 'sperm banks' where men transact big business with sperms. Critical concern

---

[15] Dieter Giesen, *Die künstliche Insemination als ethisches und rechliches Problem* (Bielefeld: Verlag Ernst und Werner Gieseking, 1962).

[16] *A.A.S.*, 41 (September 29, 1949), pp. 557 ff.

is justifiable in view of the total separation of procreation from the unitive aspect of sexuality in such instances.

In the case of artificial insemination with the husband's sperm, Pius XII is less explicit: 'One does not necessarily proscribe the use of certain artificial methods intended simply either to facilitate or to enable the natural act effected in a normal manner to attain its end.' [17] As to the limits indicated by these words, discussions have been going on ever since. Many point to the cautious expressions which suggest that the pope did not want to determine possible limits to the very last detail.

When the sperm comes from the husband and the whole marriage is lived in a climate of love, then not only is he biologically the father but there is not that total severance between the unitive and the procreative meaning of marriage. It seems that Pope Pius XII wanted, above all, to exclude a voluntary ejaculation as the means of obtaining the sperm to be used for artificial insemination. But since then, within Catholic circles, a new approach has been found relative to voluntary ejaculation which is still the clinically indicated method for obtaining sperms for fertlity tests and for diagnostic purposes.

In the past some moralists suggested the use of a slightly perforated condom, so that by depositing a portion of the seed in the vagina, the biological nature would be respected; today, this method is considered abusive and immoral. Besides, it falls short of diagnostic requirements. 'Since the spiritual aspect belongs to the nature of human sexuality, the intentionality does not only determine the goal, but also codetermines the structure of the act. Voluntary (directly intended) ejaculation for well-justified diagnostic aims therefore does not constitute ipsation.' [18] 'Experience proves that voluntary ejaculation for a diagnostic goal does not induce any syndrome of masturbatory attitudes.' [19]

---

[17] *Ibid.*, p. 561.
[18] Cf.: The declaration of the Holy Office (July 24, 1929). Denzinger-Schönmetzer 2201.
[19] M. Vodipivec, 'Samenuntersuchung,' *Lexikon für Theologie,* IX (Freiburg, 1964), p. 296.

In scanning the discussions of the last decade, we can say that on artificial insemination by the husband's sperm, various opinions are possible. There are no convincing arguments to prove either the immorality of ejaculation by the husband in view of fatherhood nor the immorality of introducing that sperm into the wife's uterus. It cannot be denied that our feelings, so deeply conditioned by tradition, rebel when faced with such an unusual problematic. However, we have to see the loftiness of the parental vocation as an essential part of marriage, and the immense joy of the husband and wife who, for years, have desired children and through this manipulation are now able to receive their own child in an atmosphere of genuine love.[20]

Artificial insemination in the strictest sense of the word is now in sight through *test-tube babies*. Fertilization of the ovum and development of the germinal cell through the initial cell stages occur outside the mother's womb with the intention of eventual implantation. The moral judgment in this case is even more complex. We must first consider the considerable risks inherent in such experimentation: how many of the fertilized eggs will perish? We are not to forget, however, the high rate of loss after *in vivo* fertilization. It may be that in the earlier experimental phases the loss will be higher, but with progress in procedural techniques, scientists might be able to reduce the risk to a minimum. Those who are convinced of 'ensoulment' at the moment of fertilization will be forced to cry 'immorality' in reference to the procedure, especially if it must be interrupted at a certain stage. In their eyes, this is homicide. However, if at the present stage of embryological science we give high probability to the opinion that individualization does not coincide with fertlization — that hominization in the full sense happens at a later stage — then experimentation at initial cell division stages cannot be called homicide. This is not yet a conclusive judgment. I express only my conviction that moral difficulties are not insurmountable as long as it appears that the risk is kept within proportionate limits. However, at this

---

[20] Chiavacci, *Rivista di teologia morale, op. cit.*, p. 14.

point of reflection, we must realize how shocking the 'desacralization' of natural processes is for people of the older generation. May I remind my reader of the *re-sacralization* which is needed today, namely, absolute respect for the dignity of the person and the right understanding of the nature of the person in his capacity to reciprocate love. The 'sacredness' of the human person has replaced the many taboos and 'sacred things.'

While the test-tube baby, under the presupposition that implantation happens at the right moment, probably does not bring any psychological risks for the child, the situation becomes quite different in the utopia of human reproduction in the 'steel womb'.[21] In this case, the embryo would be bred outside a human milieu without that intimate relationship which characterizes the dialogical character of incipient human life. The danger here is qualitatively different. Would a person produced in this loveless way not suffer great damage psychologically in the specific human capacity to reciprocate love?

Serious reservations must be expressed regarding the prospect of parthenogenesis, that is the development of the ovum without the usual fertilization by a male sperm. The offspring would receive the one parent's genetic contribution only. Would the balance of nature be upset by this practice? How would the genetic pool be affected? These points are worthy of consideration. At the present moment, however, we cannot make any final judgment as to the degree of risk if development then proceeds in the womb of the mother.

F. *Abortion*

This section on the burning issue of abortion does not claim to propose *the* Catholic position on the question. In full awareness of Catholic tradition and transient cultural facets, one must confront all the realities of the situation, including the impact

---

[21] T. Francoeur, *Utopian Motherhood* (New York: Doubleday, 1970).

of the environment, the social group and the Church. But aside
from the noteworthy traditional legacy for which I am grateful,
I owe it to all interested readers to be justly critical of those
elements of tradition that would divert from sincere and
courageous thinking.[22]

A discriminating Catholic of the post-conciliar period can
differentiate irreformable dogmas from doctrinal teachings open
to further questioning and more or less substantial changes.
Discussions pertaining to birth regulation indicate a wide range
of developments, shifts of emphasis and sharp distinctions which
were not always obvious in the past. The Catholic theology of
today is one of discernment, of critical searching for truth in
dialogue with the modern world, especially with the leaders in
related disciplines. The last few years have witnessed an increase
in the publication of critical studies on the whole problem with
numerous contributions from Catholic theologians, philosophers
and physicians.[23] Catholic moralists are no longer a monolithic
block. The need for dialogue with the modern world and the
new insights of medicine force them to reconsider closely a
number of questions.

The severe judgment of the Church relative to abortion is

---

[22] For a more thorough treatment and more extensive documentation,
the reader is referred to the chapter which I contributed (and from
which I excerpt sections of this discussion), 'A Theological Evaluation,' *The Morality of Abortion* (J.T. Noonan, Jr., ed.), (Cambridge,
Mass.: Harvard Press, 1970), pp. 123-145.

[23] With no attempt at completeness, I refer to the following studies of
Catholics who dare a fresh look:
a) F. Böckle, 'Um den Beginn des Lebens,' *Arzt und Christ,* 14
(1968), 65-73.
b) D. Callahan, *Abortion: Law, Choice and Morality* (N.Y.: Macmillan, 1970).
c) *Theological Studies,* 31 (1970):
— A.E. Hellegers, 'Fetal Development,' pp. 3-9.
— J.F. Donceel, 'Immediate Animation and Delayed Hominization,' 76-105.
— J.G. Milhaven, 'The Abortion Debate: An Epistemological
Interpretation,' 106-124.
d) J. Gründel, 'Unterbrochene Schwangerschaft. Ein moraltheolo-
gisches Tabu?,' *Theologie der Gegenwart,* 13 (1970), 202-207.

H

commonly accepted.[24] Writers differ in that some simply repeat teachings of previous popes and the common formulations of manuals while others think that the teaching of the Church might be 'susceptible to gradual development through a process of refinement'.[25] While attempting to point out cautiously what type of refinement might realistically be expected, I shall have to re-examine a few concepts.

Distinctions hinge on a number of factors: the differentiation of the zygote through its various embryonic-fetal stages, a growing understanding of human life as personal, a better grasp of the nature of the person — all call for a more precise and critical focus on the 'moral malice' of abortion. We need to distinguish the medical from the legal, and these two from the moral definition of abortion, or else indicate the substantial agreement of the three.

My discussion on the malice of abortion will be followed by a tentative tracing of direction in which further thought and refinement of doctrine may be possible and perhaps needed. The question of legal regulation will be touched upon as well as the 'art of the possible.'

1. *The malice of abortion*

Most Catholic theologians of the traditional school, in maintaining that theology is confronted by a clear and un-changeable doctrine of the ordinary magisterium, would say that there remains only to explain clearly the reasons in support of the doctrine, and to discuss complicated cases which might be termed 'indirect' abortion. According to the principle of 'double effect,' the latter can be justified in terms of a licit medical intervention for the mother's welfare. Of paramount importance, then, is a clear statement of the reasons why abortion is considered

---

[24] Cf. *The Church in the Modern World* (GS, Art 51) quoted under section D of this chapter.

[25] *The Terrible Choice* (Washington, D.C.: J.P. Kennedy Jr. Foundation, 1968), p. 88.

intrinsically evil. It will then be possible to distinguish whether or not malice is ascribable to all cases.

My position on the malice of abortion is practically identical with that of the great Protestant theologian, Paul Ramsey.[26] In spite of the distinction between abortion and infanticide, we oppose the drawing of an artificial line of moral judgment between a born and an unborn child. The child in the mother's womb is a live human person with practically equal rights before and after birth.

A consensus has been reached that the dividing line cannot be clearly drawn in relation to viability. Not only can medical skill and knowledge progress markedly to extend viability to an earlier stage, but the real difference does not lie in whether or not the fetus can live outside the womb of the mother. The fact that it cannot survive outside its natural habitat does not allow one to deprive it of the life-saving environment. Admittedly, there remain well-grounded doubts as to the moment of 'ensoulment,' animation or conception. Where earlier moralists spoke of 'ensoulment,' today's theologians prefer 'beginning of human life' or 'hominization.'

If we argue against 'abortion,' we are aware that the word does not express the same meaning or the same 'malice' where it concerns a stage of fetal development in which, according to upright convictions, a human person is not yet existent. The arguments cannot be the same when we consider ourselves faced with a person endowed with an immortal soul, or another with a most marvellous life-process groping toward hominization. Different convictions will be reflected in the diverse approaches to the problem.

In abortion, the following fundamental values are at stake: (1) the recognition of the right of each human being to the most basic conditions of life and to life itself; (2) the protection of this right to live, especially by those who have cooperated

---

[26] Paul Ramsey, 'Reference Points in Deciding About Abortion,' *The Morality of Abortion, op. cit.,* pp. 60-100.

with the creative love of God; (3) the preservation of a right understanding of motherhood; (4) the ethical standard of the physician as one who protects and cares for human life and never becomes an agent of its destruction. The vigour of the argument derives from our belief in *the dignity of each human person* created in the image and likeness of God and in man's calling to universal brotherhood in mutual love, respect and justice.

All these values come to a focal point and acquire special urgency in the family, in the relationship between mother and child, father and child. Human solidarity, the intimate dependency of the human person on the other's love and protection — never are these more strongly disclosed than during the nine months the embryo or fetus lives on the mother's bloodstream. The psychological and moral maturity of the mother, as mother, greatly affects her attitude towards the child she is bearing. It makes an enormous difference whether she considers the fetus only as 'tissue' or entertains motherly feelings towards this living being. The humanization of all mankind, the totality of human relationships cannot be dissociated from this most fundamental and life-giving relationship between the mother and the unborn child. All forms of arbitrary rationalization to justify abortion will lead to other types of alibiing about interpersonal relationships and further explosions of violence.

The power of all these arguments comes from belief in God as Creator and Redeemer of man, the only Lord over life and death: God who is love and who calls man to mutual love, respect and care.

2. *The certainty of the presuppositions of the Catholic doctrine*

Holy Scripture does not provide us with a clearcut doctrine on all the questions and solutions pertaining to abortion. It does teach the basic values on which we ground our arguments: the dignity of man, protection of innocent life, the concept of parenthood, the commandment to love. All this becomes an urgent rule of love whereby the life of our neighbour can and must be protected. There is at least a probability that the word *pharmakeia* which Paul includes in his catalogue of the fruits of self-indulgence (Gal 5 : 20) condemns abortion along with any other use of drugs for magical or inimical intentions.[27]

Whatever may be the evidence of the biblical texts, it is certain that ever since apostolic times Christianity has taken a very severe stand against abortion, equating it with homicide.[28] Like infanticide, abortion is considered a direct transgression of the commandment to love one's neighbour. In speaking about abortion, the Fathers often called it parricide, thus showing that, in their view, abortion added to the sin against life another sin against the fundamental relationship between parents and offspring.

The presupposition for condemning abortion as *homicide* or *parricide* was that the *in utero* life was believed to be a truly human life. This held only to the extent that the embryo or fetus could be considered a human person, a human being with an immortal soul. Even in the past, there was no definitive doctrine about the moment when the embryo became animated; what could be said was that already in the first weeks, it was a life-to-be, a man, under the protection of the Giver of life.

Evidently, it should make a great difference in the moral judgment passed whether one considers the embryo or fetus as already endowed with a human life, thus possessing fully the status of a person, or only a tissue or living entity on the way to becoming a human being. Jerome and Augustine were already acutely aware of this difference.[29] However, they remained very firm in disapproving of abortion whether before or after the moment of animation (not to be overlooked is the fact that they were equally severe with respect to contraception).

As long as the common convictions within the culture

---

[27] See also: Rev 9:21; 18:23; 21:8; 22:15.

[28] John T. Noonan, Jr., 'An Almost Absolute Value in History,' *The Morality of Abortion, op. cit.,* pp. 1-59.

[29] Jerome, *Epistles,* 121, 4 *Corpus Scriptorum Ecclesiasticorum Latinorum* 56, 16; Augustine, *De origine animae,* IV, 4 *Patrologiae Cursus Completus, Series Latina,* 44, 527.

strongly favoured the opinion of animation occurring in a later stage of fetal development, most theologians, while still firmly condemning abortion in general, could think that there might be grave reasons in extraordinary cases that could justify the abortion of an 'unensouled' fetus. Many theologians did indeed express such opinions without being condemned by the Church. Thomas Sanchez, who developed a detailed casuistry, could follow many previous famous theologians.[30]

Since the first centuries, the Church has issued grave sanctions against those Christians who would dare commit such a crime as abortion. When moralists dealt with those cases which, in their opinion, did not involve the malice or evil which makes abortion so grievous a sin, they concluded that these extreme cases did not fall under the sanctions of the Church.

It is interesting to consider an effort by the highest authority of the Catholic Church to legislate sanctions while ignoring this pointed dispute among the leading theologians. In the bull *Effraenatam*, Sixtus V (October 29, 1588) decreed that all penalties of canon law and secular law be applied to all those committing abortion, whatever be the age of the fetus. Absolution from excommunication was reserved to the Holy See. Even a therapeutic intervention seemed included, although the bull aimed directly at combating prostitution in Rome. Since the bull met strong opposition among moralists and canonists and did not have the hoped-for success, Gregory XIV decided that the earlier legal situation should be restored.[31]

---

[30] Sanchez declared the abortion of an 'unensouled' fetus lawful for several grave reasons, *e.g.*, after conception through adultery where this would expose not only the woman's honour but also her life. *Disputationum de matrimonii sacramento*, bk. IX, Disp. XX 8 (Viterbo 1754), vol. II, p. 171. Very interesting also is his argument in the matter of saving the life of the mother in extreme danger (*Ibid.*, Disp. XX, 9, p. 230). An impressive list of renowned Catholic moralists is quoted by Sanchez and by Laymann, *Theologia moralis*, bk. III, part III, chap. IV, 4 (Pavia, 1733), pp. 324-325.

[31] The cases under dispute, and generally the abortion of the fetus considered as yet 'unensouled' were no longer to fall under the

Throughout the centuries, theological opinions have followed closely upon those of scientists and physicians. Under the heading 'the beginning of human life,' I have discussed at length the various theories bearing on the problem of animation and individualization. Here I shall only synthesize this by saying that at this present stage of fetology, we cannot state a specific or accurate moment of hominization, although there is never any doubt of the developing process. As the fetus develops, there is an increasing degree of certainty that it has become a human being. On the other hand, there is also a growing consensus that not before implantation, and perhaps not even before the development of the basic brain structure, is individualization a full reality. Therefore, at this stage, there is a higher probability that we are not yet faced with a fully human being.

Up to the moment of complete individualization, the traditional judgment about the absolute immorality of the direct interruption of pregnancy might be modified in extreme cases of conflict of values and duties. At this point, we cannot disregard the most serious fact that during the past centuries Catholic moralists all too easily justified mass killings of fully developed men in what they termed 'just wars'. Our concern about capital punishment and our most energetic efforts to free humanity from the age-old slavery of war would become incredible if, on moral grounds, we justified abortion in the full sense of the term. However, in difficult cases and particularly during the period where individualization has most probably not happened, we seem to be entitled to refer to the traditional doctrine of conflict of duties or conflict of values. But these cases have to be clearly delineated and limited much more carefully than traditional theology limited the 'just war'.

---

sanctions. The expression with which the bull of Sixtus V was invalidated is interesting: 'the respective part should be considered as if it had never issued' (ac si eadem constitutio in huiusmodi parte numquam emanasset), *Sedes apostolica, Magnum bullarium romanum* (Luxembourg, 1942), vol. II, p. 766.

3. The Catholic position in a pluralistic society

In 1961, the Jesuit John J. Lynch deplored the professed inability of our separated brethren to understand our cogent manner of arguing about the intrinsic immorality of contraception. He thought that ecumenical dialogue demanded only a great effort to explain to them the meaning of our immutable position as an exigency of our faith,[32] though he was quite pessimistic about the possibility of convincing even the most open-minded Protestants. Since then, theological discussion has helped greatly to distinguish what is immutable in our position and what can and must be further developed and better grounded for mutual understanding.

I do not think that we can compare the discussion on abortion with that on contraception. There is however a wide area of common ground among Catholics and Protestants relative to abortion in general, even if there are different positions in difficult situations. In a 1970 joint declaration of the Catholic and Protestant hierarchy of West Germany on the duty of the state to protect the innocent life of the fetus, there is great evidence of this common ground.[33] After clear moral condemnation of abortion, the statement says, 'From the moral point of view, an exception to the principle of the inviolability of the growing life in the mother's womb can be discussed only in such cases as conflict with higher or equally high value and right, i.e., in a conflict of conscience based on such a conflict of duties.' I feel that the position of Paul Ramsey, which is very close to my own, is shared by many Protestants in all countries. Perhaps we can say that the position of another famous Protestant ethicist, James Gustafson, is at least not very far from the position of Catholic thinkers of the past which we have reviewed.[34]

My feeling is that a large area of agreement could be

---

[32] John J. Lynch, 'Notes on Moral Theology,' *Theological Studies*, 22 (1961), 255-256.

[33] The text may be found in *Herder Korrespondenz*, 25 (1971), 86-92.

[34] James M. Gustafson, 'A Protestant Ethical Approach,' *The Morality of Abortion, op. cit.*, pp. 101-122.

developed if we, on our part, were able to distinguish very carefully the essence of our doctrine from the less sure conclusions and arguments. The official position of the Catholic Church, which in most respects is well grounded, will be weakened in the eyes of Protestants and critical Catholics, especially physicians, if we fail to account clearly for the different degrees of certainty of our presuppositions, and to acknowledge the intellectual difficulties regarding troublesome cases which are now falling under the official condemnation of the Church, although, until the end of the nineteenth century, they were freely discussed.

To my knowledge, Protestant writers affirm unambiguously the same basic moral values as those on which we ground our own arguments; there is, therefore, a broad agreement about the immorality of abortion in general. Disagreement arises chiefly in reference to hard cases, where Protestants hold that, because of special circumstances, other moral values dominate in such a way that what is still called abortion does not show the specific malice of abortion. St Alphonsus Liguori asserts that *epikeia* (which frees from the particular law if there is a certain or truly probable opinion that the legislator, acting wisely, could not have intended to include such an extraordinary case in his law) can be used even in matters of *natural law* where, owing to the situation, the action would not be characterized by that malice which is the reason for the immorality asserted in the principle.[35] Following this view, Alphonsus did at least consider the probability of the opinion that the need to save the life of the mother in imminent danger of death might free the therapeutic abortion from the typical malice of abortion, though on the practical level, he favoured the safer opinion of those who were teaching that a direct intention of abortion should be excluded. But his final argument is puzzling, since he repeats twice in the context, 'why expel it (the fetus) directly since it is lawful and sufficient to do it indirectly?'[36]

---

[35] *Theologia moralis*, bk. I, treatise II, n. 201 (Ed. Gaudé, 1905), vol. I, p. 182.
[36] *Ibid.*, pp. 644, 646.

It is true that since the end of the last century the Holy See has moved further towards eliminating milder opinions which earlier were proposed by renowned Catholic moralists. The Catholic theologian will manifest loyal adherence to these decisions. However, a scientific attitude open to new insights, concern for credibility and for our earnest ecumenical dialogue force him to discuss important distinctions: What is the essential and abiding part of the official teaching and what is a special pastoral aspect or a less convincing application? To what extent is part of a doctrine, presented in the name of 'natural law,' binding for all times if the arguments given by the magisterium are not fully convincing and if theology remains unable to supply more persuasive reasons? Finally, how can the magisterium maintain a part of its official teaching if, in view of new scientific data, the arguments are not fully cogent and no longer convincing? If it is really a matter of natural law, then it is chiefly a question of human experience, reflection and shared insights.

I wish to state clearly my own approach to the problem. If I argue about questions which seem to have been decided by the magisterium, though not in an irreformable way, I do not recommend my tentative opinion as one to be followed in practice, except for those cases in which the arguments are fully compelling or a new common opinion is taking shape. I insist that the presumption is in favour of the teaching office of the magisterium. A doubt by some theologian does not invalidate the official position; later discussions may even strengthen it and bring forth more convincing arguments. It is in this attitude that I propose some thoughts about possible directions for a refinement of the actual teaching of the Catholic Church on abortion. On some points, there is evidence of a newly emergent opinion.

4. *A sharper distinction between abortion and contraception*

In the past, contraception and abortion were somehow put on the same plane as crimes against nature and against the pro-creative function of sexuality. The result was a blurring of the specific malice and basis for the immorality of abortion. An insufficient effort of this kind was understandable at a time when moralists accepted the opinion that the fetus of the male was animated on the fortieth day after fertilization and that of the female on the eightieth day, and when they sharply distinguished the abortion of 'ensouled' and 'unensouled' fetuses.

The encyclical *Casti connubii* is probably the most classical official text condemning contraception and abortion with almost equal severity. The encyclical was specifically worded and directed to oppose the teaching of the Lambeth Conference about contraception, and was inspired by a widespread fear that contempt for life expressed in a contraceptive attitude would not only cause serious demographic problems (imbalance between old and young) but also destroy the very ideal of parenthood and conjugal chastity.[37] There was evidently a strong conviction that the tendency towards abortion could not be conquered without first fighting the source of the evil, the contraceptive attitude. Again, the want of critical distinctions failed to differentiate contraception *per se* from a responsible transmission of life.

Between the encyclical *Casti connubii* (1930) and the teaching of the Second Vatican Council lie thirty-five years of rich experience, of sociological and psychological studies and reflection. It is no wonder, then, that the teaching of the Second Vatican Council shows an acute awareness of the total difference between birth regulation by contraception (which can be motivated by responsible parenthood) and abortion.

If rigoristic formulations of the teaching on contraception and even more inflexible pastoral application of that teaching were among the causes of an increase in abortions in some groups of the Catholic population (for example, in Latin America), then there arises an urgent need for more careful differentiation of actions so totally different as abortion and contraception. If a contraceptive attitude is one of the chief causes of abortion, a conscientious use of the best possible methods of birth regulation in the spirit of responsible parenthood can remove many temptations to resort to such criminal means.

---

[37] Pius XI, *Casti Connubii, Acta Apostolicae Sedis,* 22 (1930), pp. 539-592.

The Church's condemnation of abortion becomes fully credible only if, simultaneously, all possible efforts are made to eliminate the causes of the problem. These efforts should include truly pastoral wording of the Church's doctrine as well as all kinds of social action in favour of those who lie especially exposed to the danger of 'resolving' their hard problems by abortion.

In some instances, science and ethics are incapable as yet of determining with certainty whether a certain means is contraceptive only or abortifacient. Such is the case with the intrauterine device which most probably serves to block implantation of the morula. Similarly, the 'morning-after pill' is taken in order to ensure non-implantation. Although we are not sure whether there is human life in the full sense at this early stage of development, these means cannot simply be equated with contraception. At the present stage of scientific and ethical insights, not only can they not be endorsed as means of birth regulation but must be discussed under the heading of abortion.

5. Clearer distinctions of the malice of abortion

Traditional moral theology sharply distinguished direct from indirect abortion, condemning the first and condoning the latter. However, indirect abortion can be lawful only on condition that it is not an abortion in the moral sense, that is, that it does not bear the moral malice of abortion.

Many moralists of the past centuries spoke of indirect abortion in a very broad sense. For instance, Augustine Lehmkuhl was still asserting in 1888 that an abortion (an expulsion) of a nonviable fetus to save the life of the mother would scarcely be 'a direct abortion in a theological sense, any more than yielding a plank in a shipwreck to a friend is direct killing of one's self.' [38]

---

[38] August Lehmkuhl, *Theologia moralis* (Freiburg im Br., 7th ed., 1893), vol. I, n. 841, p. 500. Only in the 9th edition (1898, vol. I, n. 841 and 844) did he change his position. But it remains uncertain whether he was really convinced of the necessity to change his opinion. He writes in n. 844 (9th ed., vol. I., p. 502): 'It is said, in accordance with the judgment of the Holy Office that my earlier opinion cannot be followed in practice (tuto).'

Earlier moralists justifying 'indirect abortion' applied this teaching in one way or another to almost all cases where the chief and decisive intention was directed towards another exalted good such as the health and life of the mother. Depriving the fetus of life was then only the secondary effect of the intention and action: secondary in so far as it was not willed in itself. In accordance with the principle of double effect, there also had to be a very evident proportion between the risk to fetal life and the motives justifying the action.

It was chiefly out of pastoral concern that the Holy See took up a position which was against any therapeutic abortion. The rigid stance came in response to the concern of several bishops who had informed the Roman authorities that ' a way had been found to abort the fetus by means which did not directly tend to its killing in the mother's womb but to its expulsion, so that it would die as soon as it came to light.' [39]

Faced with a multitude of people either unable to distinguish or else inclined to all-too-subtle distinctions, the pastoral solicitude of Pius XI and Pius XII led them to condemn vehemently any kind of direct abortion and to declare the absolute inviolability of life, allowing no exception.[40] One of the beneficial results was that Catholic gynecologists, because of the necessity for extraordinary effort, made special contributions to the saving of life both of the mother and of the fetus.

But the question of what constitutes *direct* and *indirect* abortion was not settled in Catholic moral theology. The standard cases of ectopic pregnancy and of a cancerous uterus found approval by the majority of Catholic moralists. The physician was surely allowed to perform all the medically accepted operations with the standard procedures in so far as they appeared necessary and urgent to remedy an acute, hazardous, morbid

---

[39] Denzinger-Schönmetzer, *Enchiridion Symbolorum*, 32nd ed. (Freiburg/Breisgau and New York, 1963), no. 3298.
[40] Pius XI, *Casti connubii*, *A.A.S.*, pp. 262-265.
Pius XII, Address to the Catholic Society of Midwives (October 29, 1951), *Acta Apostolicae Sedis*, 43 (1951), pp. 838 ff.

condition of the expectant mother, even if these medical interventions entailed a probable or even certain danger to the fetal
life as an undesired and indirect consequence. The condition
was always that no real probability existed to save both the
mother and the unborn child.

The distinction between 'direct' and 'indirect' abortion has
sometimes resulted in mechanical or too literal applications. A
gynecologist tells of a typical case: 'I was once called upon to
perform an operation on a woman in the fourth month of
pregnancy, to remove a benign uterine tumour. On the womb,
there were numerous very thin and fragile varicose veins which
bled profusely, and attempts to suture them only aggravated the
bleeding. Therefore, in order to save the woman from bleeding to
death, I opened the womb and removed the fetus. Thereupon
the uterus contracted, the bleeding ceased, and the woman's life
was saved. I was proud of what I had achieved, since the uterus
of this woman, who was still childless, was undamaged and she
could bear other children. But I had to find out later from a
noted moralist that although I had indeed acted in good faith,
what I had done was, in his eyes, *objectively* wrong. I would
have been allowed to remove the bleeding uterus with the fetus
itself, he said, but was not permitted to interrupt the pregnancy
while leaving the womb intact. He informed me that my intervention constituted an immoral termination of pregnancy, even
though the purpose was to save the mother, whereas the other
way would have been a lawful direct intention (*prima intentio*)
and action to save life, as in the case of a cancerous uterus. For
him, preservation of the woman's fertility and in some cases,
preservation of the marriage itself, played no decisive *rôle*.' [41]

My judgment of a similar case would follow a line of
reasoning quite different from that of the moralist mentioned.
The malice of abortion is an attack on the right of the fetus to
live. Since the doctor in this situation can determine with great

---

[41] H. Kramann, 'Umstrittene Heilmethoden in der Gynekologie,' *Arzt
und Christ*, 5 (1959), 202 ff. See my book, *The Law of Christ*,
Vol. III (Westminster, Md.: Newman Press, 1966), p. 212.

moral certainty that there is no chance for both the mother and the fetus to survive without his 'direct' intervention, he accepts the only chance to protect and serve life which Divine Providence has left to him. He saves the life of the mother while he does not truly deprive the fetus of its right to live since it could not possibly survive in the event of the doctor's failure to save the mother's life. Moreover, the preservation of the mother's fertility is an additional service to life.

As we already distinguish in abortion (or interruption of a pregnancy) between a *medical* and a *legal* sense, I propose the further distinction of a *moral* sense. Morally-speaking, abortion would designate all cases bearing the characteristic malice which justifies our severe condemnation of it. Practically, this solution would not go much further than the casuistic solutions of those moralists who undertook the problem only with the principle of double effect and indirect action, but my way of arguing seems to be — at least in somes cases — less artificial.

I do not, however, deny the value of the common distinctions of 'direct' and 'indirect.' They allow, for example, a quite reasonable solution in the case of ectopic pregnancy. The reason for terminating a pregnancy cannot be the fetus as such, but only a dangerous development such as a pathological pregnancy in the Fallopian tube. But even in this case, my own way of arguing seems to be simpler and more persuasive. The physician should do his best to preserve the fetus in the case of ectopic conception but as soon as it becomes certain — as is normally the case — that intervention is mandatory to save the mother, and there is no chance to save both by waiting, the intervention does not truly deprive the fetus of the right to live, since it has already no chance to survive. The fact that the biological death occurs some days earlier than if the physician allowed both to die does no harm to the right of the fetus since this very slight shortening of fetal existence does not deprive it of any personal activity.

6. *Human being defined*

Hitler destroyed hundreds of thousands of people because he considered them to be 'unfit for life.' His sole criterion was man's utility for the type of economic and political society he wished to bring about. Little did he understand that the patience, loving acceptance and suffering of the afflicted can enrich the whole of mankind. But a person's value cannot be a function of social usefulness and fitness. Whether useful for earthly purposes or not, the life of the human person is always sacred.

I cannot, therefore, see any truly moral justification for the interruption of pregnancy because of a probability that the child might be defective (e.g., as in the case of thalidomide children). Supposing that in the near future, man would reach moral certainty that up to a certain developmental stage the embryo is not yet endowed with *human* life (is not yet a person), and assuming that the developing diagnostic procedures could detect fetal anomalies before that stage, there would be a margin for responsible intervention based on rigid eugenic criteria. Teilhard de Chardin seems to indicate this hypothesis. 'So far we have certainly allowed our race to develop at random, and we have given too little thought to the question of what medical and moral factors must replace the crude forces of natural selection should we suppress them. In the course of the coming centuries, it is indispensable that a nobly human form of eugenics, on a standard worthy of our personalities, should be discovered and developed.' [42] I am convinced that in the eyes of Teilhard the killing of a human being would not be a 'nobly human form of eugenics.' But Teilhard de Chardin did face the responsible prospect of genetic engineering and a courageous approach to new questions: 'With the discovery of genes we shall soon be able to control the mechanism of organic heredity.' [43]

Quite different from proposing the killing of a human person is the modern moralist's forced confrontation with the following question: Is a totally deformed fetus that is lacking even the biological substratum for any expression of truly human life, still to be considered a person? Is it wholly clear that we must preserve, with tremendous effort and hurt, a biological life born

---

[42] Teilhard de Chardin, *The Phenomenon of Man, op. cit.,* p. 282.
[43] Teilhard de Chardin, *The Phenomenon of Man, op. cit.,* p. 250.

of a human mother if there is not and never will be the slightest expression of humanity? Would it be an abortion in the full moral sense if the doctor, after a clear diagnosis of such a total deformation (*e.g.*, anencephaly) were to interrupt a pregnancy?

I am not sure whether this question can find a safe and certain answer at the present stage of discussion,[44] but it is worth considering, since our concern is not just for biological life but for *human* life. In no way does the question suggest a justification of euthanasia. Rather, in my opinion, the problem is analogous to that of whether we should keep organs alive after confirmation of 'brain death' (to be treated in the next chapter). Though a person may suffer deeply in the last days or month of his life, it can still be a blessed human experience; there can be most important personal manifestations of faith, trust, patience and gratitude. On the other hand, I do not see any need for *artificially* maintaining the biological life of an adult person or of a child for days and months if there is no hope whatsoever that this person will regain consciousness or be capable of any personal manifestation.[45] There is, however, an essential difference between killing and allowing a human being to die in dignity. Our question, once more, is different: in certain extreme cases of abnormality, are we faced with a human being when there is no bodily substratum for personhood?

---

[44] Ruff, *Stimmen der Zeit*, 181 (1968), pp. 331-335. Following other moralists, Alphonsus Liguori responds to the question about the abortion of a totally deformed fetus that has no chances of survival: 'As Sporer and Holzman rightly assert, there must be made an exception in the case of a corrupted fetus, because if it is deformed to an extent that it is no longer apt to be ensouled it is no more a fetus, but just a putrid substance.' *Theologia moralis*, III, treatise II, Doubt IV, n. 394, (Ed. Gaudé), vol. I, p. 645. Of course, the problem poses itself to these moralists in a somewhat different perspective because their casuistic solutions are based on the rather oversimplified theory of successive animation. Ruff gives a modern version of these theories.

[45] Cardinal Michele Pellegrino, 'Questioni deontologiche nella pratica cardiologica,' *Minerva Medica*, 59 (1968), 1594-1596.

I

7. *Moral principles and pastoral counselling*

Gustafson has made a major contribution to the discussions of situation ethics by distinguishing the different levels of discourse.[46] One should clearly realize the level at which dialogue is to proceed. Most of Gustafson's article on abortion remains on what he calls the second level, the reflective question of a person asking, 'What ought I do in this situation?' After being raped, a woman seeks advice; she and her counsellor will discuss the question in a discourse essentially on the same level.[47]

Up to this point, my discussion has been at the 'third or ethical level' where questions are raised about general rules or considerations that would justify a particular moral judgment. Catholic theology has a long tradition of distinguishing clearly the level at which one confronts a problem; for instance, we distinguish the level of moral theology from that of pastoral counselling. The approaches differ somewhat but mine can be compared to Gustafson's.

On the level of pastoral counselling, a Catholic moralist might reach the same conclusion and even come to an almost identical manner of friendly discourse as Gustafson. Pastoral and medical prudence look not only to general principles but also to the art of the possible. By realistically seeking the next possible step to be taken by a person in this concrete situation, the pastoral effort of the moral theologian does not betray his own 'objective' principles since the whole of moral life is characterized by the 'law of growth,' by the need for a constant but gradual conversion. The milder tradition of moral and pastoral theology expresses an important aspect of this dynamic approach in its discourse on 'invincible ignorance.'

Invincible ignorance should not be interpreted in a merely intellectualized sense but more in the light of a theory of

---

[46] James F. Gustafson, 'Context Versus Principles. A Displaced Debate in Christian Ethics,' *The Harvard Theological Review*, 58 (1965), 171-202.

[47] J.F. Gustafson, 'Protestant Ethical Approach,' in *The Morality of Abortion, op. cit.,* pp. 101-122.

conscience which emphasizes the existential wholeness of man. Invincible ignorance pertains to the inability of a person to 'realize' a moral obligation. Because of his previous experience, psychological impasses and the whole context of his life, a person is unable to cope with a certain moral imperative. His intellectual inefficiency in grasping the values behind a certain command is often deeply rooted in existential difficulties. Are we not all in the condition of the disciples to whom the Lord says: 'There is still much that I could say to you but the burden would be too great for you now' (Jn 16: 12)? According to the very different stature and situation of people, this can be the case not only with regard to the highest ideals and ultimate commandments of the Gospel, but also with respect to a concrete, existential understanding of a prohibitive moral norm.

Alphonsus Liguori expresses the basic principle of moral counselling in cases of invincible ignorance in the following way: 'The more common and true opinion teaches that the confessor can and must refrain from admonition and leave the penitent in good faith whenever he is confronted with an invincible error, whether in matter of human law or in matter of divine law, if prudence tells him that an admonition would not do any good but rather harm the penitent.' [48] The main concern of pastoral counselling must always be the conscience of the person and not abstract rules. Alphonsus explains that 'the reason is that there must be more care to avoid the danger of a formal sin than to avoid that of a material sin. God punishes only the formal sin, since he takes only this as an offence.' [49]

In his moral discourse, Gustafson cites the example of a woman who seeks counsel after a heinous rape committed against her by her ex-husband and a group of scoundrels. I had earlier explained my approach to a similar case; I then expressed myself on the 'third level,' as a moralist stating an opinion about objective norms. I wrote: 'In cases of rape, it is morally permis-

---

[48] *Theologia moralis,* bk. VI, treatise IV, n. 610 (Ed. Gaudé, 1905), vol. III, p. 634.
[49] *Praxis confessarii,* chapter 1, n. 8 (exceptions to principle included).

sible to cleanse away the sperm, which is considered to be an extension of the initial act of aggression. Abortion, however, is not allowed if conception has already taken place. It has not been adjudged that the fetus, which would not have been formed except for the presence of the 'aggressive' sperm, is itself an 'aggressor.' [50]

Then, turning to the level of pastoral counselling I continued: 'Nevertheless, we must recognize that although the fetus is innocent, the girl is likewise innocent. We can therefore understand her revulsive feeling that this is not 'her' child, not a child that she is, in justice, required to bear. We must, however, *try to motivate her* to consider the child with love because of its subjective innocence, and to bear it in suffering up to birth, whereupon she may consider her enforced maternal obligation fulfilled and may give over the child to a religious or governmental agency, after which she would try to resume her life with the sanctity that she will undoubtedly have achieved through the great sacrifice and suffering. If, owing to the psychological effects of her traumatic experience, she is unable to accept this counsel, it is possible that we may have to leave her in 'invincible ignorance.' Her own salvation may depend on it because of her near despair. If she has already yielded to the violent temptation to rid herself as completely as possible of the effects of her experience, we can leave the judgment of the degree of her sin to a merciful God and try to build up her willingness to integrate both her suffering and her fault with the sufferings and sins of the world that Christ took upon himself on the cross.' [51]

While it is true that this mode of expression differs from the style and approach of Gustafson, since my references are within the frame of reference of the specific Catholic tradition of pastoral theology, I do not perceive the two positions to be irreconcilable in essence. I did not write that the confessor or

---

[50] B. Häring, *Shalom: Peace* (New York: Farrar-Straus-Giroux, 1967), p. 181.
[51] B. Häring, *Shalom: Peace, op. cit.,* p. 182.

counsellor should first impart the moral principles. A pastoral attempt at motivation excludes an immediate presentation of abstract principles and consequent imperatives. Proper motivation is the first imperative. The counsellor will then be in a better position to assess the exent to which a person can accept the appeal for a heroic solution.

My pastoral concern however would never express itself in such terms as to advise abortion of the fetus; neither would I give a nod of approval to the woman's decision to seek an abortion. But in the course of pastoral counselling, I would refrain from all rigid judgment and show respect for the convictions and conscience of the person. I would not pursue the question once it had become evident that the woman could not bear the burden of the pregnancy. The decision remains hers always, not mine.

Similarly, I fail to see that a physician can be charged with the malice of abortion if the rape victim cannot be induced to keep the fetus and if therefore, he is regretfully obliged to accept what, in his eyes, is the best possible solution. This is especially so when the physician is firmly convinced that the fetus has not yet reached the stage of final 'individualization.'

8. *The morality of legislation*

Legislation and approved customs have played a large part in the formation of conscience and in the motivation of people in homogeneous and closed cultural groups and especially in the less developed sectors of those societies. The encyclical *Casti connubii* evidently addressed itself to such societies, and consequently did not come to a clear distinction between morality *per se* and legislation; it seems, then, that for Pius XI each sin calls for a penal sanction. He admonished the legislator, 'to take into account what is determined by the divine law and by the legislation of the Church, and to proceed with penal sanctions against those who have sinned. For people are thinking that whatever is allowed by civil legislation or not subject to penal sanctions may also be allowed according to the moral law; or they may put it into practice even against their conscience, since they do not fear God and would not have to fear anything from human legislation.' [52] Such an approach to penal law does not fit into the vision adopted by the Declaration of the Second Vatican Council on religious liberty nor does it take into account the new situation of modern society.

In a pluralistic society one of the most urgent duties of the churches and of humanist ethicists is to contribute to the formation of a mature conscience. Every responsible person must be clearly aware that true morality and penal sanctions — or the absence of penal sanctions — lie on two quite different levels. Legislation or custom alone must not be allowed to determine our moral judgment; the Church has to instruct the faithful that conscience is to be formed by the Gospel and by insight into moral values. For many cultures, it is true that the combination of law with custom provides one of the easier sources of accessibility to moral insight, but in a pluralistic society the rôle of this source has dwindled. As a result, a shift towards direct personal insight into the levels and urgencies of moral values is most necessary for all. We should consider this shift as offering greater impetus towards maturity and depth, although it may also entail dangers for weaker personalities.

Modern pluralistic states, especially the United States of America, Great Britain and Canada, have become less and less able to enforce the penalties against abortion, particularly where citizens and even Christian ethicists are no longer in agreement about the hierarchy of values and its principal applications. Under such circumstances the Church's undue emphasis on a strengthening of penal legislation could sacrifice an opportunity to work for a deeper formation of the consciences of the faithful. The present discussions should lead to an awakening of the conscience of many about their responsibilities in confronting and resolving not only the issue of abortion but also other urgent issues.

The formation of conscience demands good and absolutely honest argument, including a fairly clear distinction between the

---

[52] Pius XI, *Casti connubii, op. cit.,* p. 589.

existence of an official teaching and reasoning relative to moral values. Only within the Church itself is the existence of doctrinal teaching a strong argument; in dialogue with others, it has little bearing. Since legislation in a modern democratic state depends greatly on public opinion, all who are convinced of the need for certain legislation to protect the innocent life of the fetus should give attention to the art of influencing public opinion by appropriate methods and arguments.

A campaign for a better-informed public and for laws protecting the life of the unborn child becomes credible, honest and effective to the extent that all genuine opportunities for social assistance in difficult situations are available and used to the utmost. Since protection by penal legislation is weakening, there should be more intelligent efforts on our part to enlighten public opinion on the whole issue. We could well do with more active leadership in creating and sustaining initiatives designed to remove the chief causes of abortion. A combined teaching-action programme would be likely to provide untapped resources of motivation.

As far as legislation is concerned, it should be discussed chiefly in terms of the common good, justice towards the weak, protection of those basic values without which society would be exposed to great risks of self-destruction. It cannot be the task of a pluralistic state to protect the religious teaching of a church where this does not coincide with the generally acknowledged common good of that society. If we argue on the basis of natural law, this can be effective only to the extent that we give, in addition to the official teaching of ecclesiastical authority, reasons and motives that could be convincing to sincere and intelligent people who are not under the authority of the Church.

I am not at all enthusiastic about the Abortion Act of Great Britain of October 27, 1967. While there is a conscience clause so that no one can be forced to participate in any abortion if he has conscientious objection to it, I strongly disagree with the restriction in this clause which deprives of its benefits anyone who 'has a duty to participate in treatment which is necessary to save the life or to prevent grave permanent injury to the physical or mental health of a pregnant woman.' This is most deplorable since it may be interpreted as obliging, for example, a Catholic doctor, under penal sanctions, to act against his own conscience and terminate pregnancies by procedures which can be judged as directly abortifacient.

On the other hand, if it is a matter of discussing the qualities of the legislation *as* legislation, I do not find the following type of discussion very helpful: 'Mother and child have an equal right to life and no action is moral that favours the life of one against that of another. No Catholic, or indeed anyone — for the law of God governs all men — may take part in this type of abortion. . . . Direct abortion is always against the positive and natural law of God. Indirect abortion may sometimes be permitted for a sufficiently grave reason.'[53] I do not deny the basic value which, at least for Catholic theologians, is behind this argument, but it does not reach the partners of the dialogue and does not seem to be the point of legislation as such.

I would argue strongly against the restriction, but along the following lines: One of the great values and foundations of a religiously pluralistic state is respect for the moral and religious convictions of loyal and serious citizens. There is no good reason, in view of the common good and the fundamental right of all citizens, to disregard the upright moral conviction of many Catholics who, on this point, abide by the official teaching of their Church. This disregard for the conscience of Catholic doctors and others who share their convictions is the more deplorable because the restriction in the conscience clause is so worded that it might invite pressure against doctors for not interrupting a pregnancy. This law seems also to contradict the common practice of modern states not to encourage people to invoke legal processes against conscientious physicians.

Any state preparing new legislation on abortion should study with great care the foreseeable impact on the common good, on respect for another person's life, and on all other values that

---

[53] Peter Flood, 'The Abortion Act 1967,' *Clergy Review* (January, 1968), 46.

could be affected by changes under consideration; but this is not the duty of legislators alone. It is likewise the responsibility of leading members of the Church, of enlightened citizens and of ethicists who wish to make concrete suggestions about the content of a law, to study at all levels the matter of probable consequences. Besides, there always remains the 'art of the possible' in the best conceivable direction.

Chapter 7

THE DEATH OF MAN

The abstract notion of death may be of academic interest in the medical school but the reality of death is what confronts the practitioner as he goes about his daily hospital rounds or meets his patients in consultation. University professors may nobly fulfil their pedagogical *rôle* by dispensing anatomical-physiological knowledge to their students relative to the concomitants of death, and may even rest content to accept and present a biological view of death as expiration. The medical practitioner cannot operate within such narrow confines; without an organismic approach to life and death, he would fail in his mission.

Physicians in private practice spend most of their working hours with persons in failing health, with dying patients and their relatives. A patient's implicit trust in his physician becomes a wish that he stand by at the hour of death. A patient's many queries about the odds for the prolongation of his life or about an impending death compel the physician to transcend his *rôle* as servant of biological life. He is then called to share his convictions in relation to a holistic understanding of human existence. In facing so often the death of others, the physician will not preserve his own balance and health short of searching with his

120

patients for the whole import of death. 'The more the physician
becomes humane, in the full sense of human, bringing his medical
service and medical ethos to completion, the more his patient's
question, "What is death?" will be that of the physician
himself.'[1]

The discussion in this chapter will cover the meaning of
death, the physician's task as he interacts with a dying patient
and his family, the new arguments relative to the moment of
death and, in that context, the prolongation of life, resuscitation
measures, transplantation, and finally, euthanasia.

A. *The meaning of death*

Death is a multi-faceted phenomenon. Not only does man's
quest for the significance of his ultimate earthly experience vary
in approach — biological, philosophical, sociological or theological — but each person apprehends his own death in a unique
way. The physician serves patients of varied beliefs whose
diverse world-views result in divergent interpretations of the
phenomenon of death. Variegations and nuances are found within
the same church or religion and are reflected in different
thoughts and attitudes relative to the 'ebb of life,' 'passing away'
and bereavement. This is to be expected since the mystery of
death surpasses in depth any particular interpretation or explanation. The most definitive differential, however, obtains from
the patient himself, in whether or not he has the courage to face
this most awesome personal mystery in full sincerity.

Does Christian faith have anything to contribute to the
understanding of death? The message of the Gospel offers no
rationalistic explanations of either life or death; like that of the
rest of scripture, its vantage point is that of salvation. Death is
presented as an ambassador of redemption or of judgment,
depending on the situation and life-choice of the person, that is,

---

[1] Karl Rahner, 'Gedanken über das Sterben,' *Arzt und Christ*, 15
(1969), 28.

depending on whether he chose dedication or egotism and superficiality. The biblical message addresses us existentially in terms of an appeal to vigilance here and now. Those who, at each decisive moment, override their egotism and open themselves to the true meaning of life know that their death experience will be the final momentous decision. Their attitude of generous acceptance liberates them from self-centred concerns and uncovers to them the wealth hidden in the last opportunity for a loving 'yes'.

The oft-discussed question of whether, without original sin, physical death would have ensued is not a specifically theological question. The 'death' that came into the world through sin is that existential plight of man who has either refused to probe the meaning of life or has rejected it. It is the despair of nothingness and meaninglessness, the repudiation of true significance in both life and death. For the sinner death becomes the final event of alienation. He is overanxious and frustrated because his faith reminds him of his failure to live truly his own life of Christian solidarity. His apprehensiveness is the result of sin.

On the cross, Jesus shares the grief and suffering of the dying because he bears the burden of all his brethren. He is the Lamb of God who takes upon himself the sin of the world, that is, the sinfulness of mankind as a whole with all its consequences. But he transforms death into the greatest manifestation of trust in the Father and love for all men by making it a wholly salvific event. Those who believe in Christ's passion, death and resurrection gain a new vision of death. No longer does it appear as a curse chastening sinful mankind but as a link in the liberating history of salvation through solidarity in Christ.

Above all, scripture depicts death as the harvest of an existential rejection of life's meaning through a choice of sinfulness, or as the moment of consummate unity with Christ and trust in God. This fact is further clarified in the Gospel of St John: 'If a man has faith in me, even though he die, he shall come to life; and no one who is alive and has faith shall ever die' (Jn 11: 25-26). 'The believer possesses eternal life. I am the bread of life . . . which a man may eat, and never die. . . . If anyone eats this bread he shall live forever' (Jn 6: 47-51; also Jn 6: 59). This astonishing message of salvation is expressed essentially and succinctly in the death of Christ, the great sign and event of saving solidarity, the greatest happening in the history of liberation. 'It was clearly fitting that God for whom and through whom all things exist should, in bringing many sons to glory, make the leader who delivers them perfect through sufferings. . . . The children of a family share the same flesh and blood; and so he too shared ours, so that through death he might break the power of him who had death at his command, that is, the evil one; and might liberate those who, through fear of death, had all their lifetime been in servitude' (Heb 2: 10-15).

Christ suffered physically but he went beyond bodily pain to assume the profound suffering of dismay and anguish in the hour of death. He thus overcame death felt as something meaningless and redeemed it through unbounded trust and forgiveness. 'In the days of his earthly life he offered up prayers and petitions, with loud cries and tears, to God who was able to deliver him from death. Because of his humble submission his prayer was heard' (Heb 5: 7) Not only was Christ delivered from the grave but all who, through him, open themselves trustingly to his saving solidarity will be delivered from that death which marks participation in the collective alienation of egotists. For them life will never be absurd, nor will death be a catastrophic ending to a meaningless life; for the saving event of Christ's life-death-resurrection transforms death into life's greatest opportunity. Instead of a futile and despairing disjunction with life, it becomes the incomparable breakthrough to life everlasting.

The thought of death may still be repugnant to the believer because of its physical distress, mental anguish and temporary separation from those he loves; yet, the Christian can join with Paul in desiring, 'I want the old body stripped off; rather, our desire is to have the new body put on over it, so that our mortal part may be absorbed into life immortal' (II Cor 5: 4). Through faith in redemption, the believer utters a firm 'yes' to life but without seeing death as inimical to true life. 'What I should

like is to depart and be with Christ; that is better by far; but
for your sake there is greater need for me to stay on in the body'
(Phil 1: 23-24).

For the Christian, death is neither a flight from the body
into the rarefied air of 'pure spirits' as suggested by much of
the Hellenistic tradition nor an alienation from bodily reality.
It is hope for the fullness of personal life, faith in the resurrection of the body and in the transfiguration of the whole person.
It holds the promise of unity with the whole of creation, and
therefore includes hope for a new heaven and a new earth, a
transformation which goes beyond all the experiences of present
faith and love.

Will this transfiguration of the whole person occur at once
through the purifying fire of encounter with the holy God? Or
is it so totally linked to the final metamorphosis of the whole
world that it will happen only at the end of days, at the
parousia? The Johannine vision of life, death and judgment
seems to suggest that, with Christ and Mary, all those who have
reached fullness of love in this life will immediately be transfigured
into a spiritual body. This differs markedly from becoming a
pure spirit or a separated soul.[2]

Decisively important is the total vision of man in the history
of salvation. Throughout his life the believer values each decision
as preparatory for the ultimate one; on his death-bed, he will
either definitively accept God's design in absolute trust and
hope or else settle for meaninglessness and despair in a last
rebellion. The Christian physician cannot be indifferent to the
believer's outlook on life, death and the hereafter. Even for the
doctor who does not share his patient's religious beliefs, it is of
paramount importance that he be cognizant of the hope and faith
of his believing patients.

No one knows better than physicians and nurses how
differently people react in the face of death. Not only are they
contrasted in their suffering and endurance, anguish or serenity,

---

[2] Cf.: Ladislaus Boros, *The Mystery of Death* (New York: Herder
and Herder, 1965).

but they differ most in their view of death; they either transcend themselves in total trust or yield in awe and dread to a final refusal of meaning.

B. *The doctor and the moribund patient*

The physician stands forever on the side of life, waging a battle against death with the full strength of his competence and commitment. His professional combat tactics and whatever supportive assistance he brings to the moribund person will depend on how he and his patient interpret the experience of death. The physician will not relent in his efforts to inspire or strengthen the patient's will-to-live and to nurture the hope of recovering health, since hope is a potent factor in the fight against death.

1. *The fullness of freedom*

Human history in general and the life history of each person are essentially chronicles of freedom. Medical assistance to the moribund assumes value to the extent that it inserts itself consciously into this history of freedom. The physician's endeavour centres on promoting that degree of consciousness, that psychosomatic condition which fosters calmness and peace for the patient in an ambience conducive to reflection, openness and freedom. The example and advice of the doctor and the nurse guide the patient's relatives and friends as they try to harmonize loving concern, trust, truthfulness and authentic peace in order to maximize the patient's exercise of freedom. The doctor will, of course, do his utmost to alleviate that pain which would be likely to restrict the ailing person's proper use of freedom at the last and most decisive moment of his life.

To a great extent the convictions of the doctor find expression in his whole professional behaviour. The physician should realize how much the patient's understanding and acceptance of death depend on his treatment and overall attitude. Besides acting in the fundamental perspective of the maturation of freedom until the last moment of conscious life, the doctor will assist the patient in achieving a *peaceful death*.[3] Since the anguish of death is its greatest terror, it should be defeated. Abiding by the criteria of freedom and peace, pain is to be relieved as much as possible. In the strength of its own autonomy, the medical action thus inserts itself into the redemptive meaning of death.

2. *A spirited quest for meaning*

The courage to confront impending death peacefully marks the culmination of personal freedom. The patient relies on the physician's magnanimous efforts to sustain his will-to-live and simultaneously to inspire confidence in face of the prospect of death. The patient gains in peacefulness and moral strength if his battle for life finds him ready to face death instead of desperately struggling against it. In this respect, much depends on the attitude of the physician and his personal view of life and death. If for him a patient's death simply represents a professional battle lost, then his bearing will do little to help the patient achieve the hoped-for serenity and balance.

A famous physician writes: 'Not only for the dying patient but also for the doctor does a strong faith generate an intensification of freedom. It allows the physician a full commitment to life without that obsession which considers death as the greatest of all evils, since we consider death as belonging to the fullness of life. The free acceptance of death is the only real chance to get out of that "death" which seems to destroy all our strength, a last opportunity to assert our freedom.'[4] Not infrequently will the doctor and his patient search together for the meaning of death, accepting patiently the question's burden of what it may finally mean to them without obtaining an immediate response. Theology cannot deny the value of such a sincere quest. It may

---

[3] Cf.: P.F. Regan, 'The Dying Patient and His Family,' *Journal of the American Medical Association,* 192 (May, 1965), 82.

[4] R. Kautzky, 'Der Arzt vor dem Phänomen des Todes,' *Arzt und Christ,* 15 (1969), 138.

be precisely in this sincerity and courage to keep on searching that man transcends himself in the direction of God.

The readiness to probe and the strength to accept the meaning of one's suffering or death are unique gifts of God which proclaim the mystery of death and resurrection and reveal its power for those who open themselves in faith. This grace is intended and signified by the sacrament of the anointing of the sick. The patient's calmness and inner peace which often follow in its wake can be a healing and life-saving adjunct to medical efforts. We need only think of heart infarct cases where serenity and peace of mind are decisive restorative factors. The same holds true for many other ailments. However, the greatest of gifts is that of optimal freedom in the acceptance of death.

3. The patient's right to truth

For physicians throughout the ages, one of the weightiest questions has centred on their responsibility and enlightened initiative in informing a dying patient about the seriousness of his situation. No stereotyped, casuistic solution can be advanced to govern all instances. The physician needs great empathy and prudence in assessing the most appropriate way of broaching the subject to each patient. Routine must be thoroughly excluded. The doctor's vast medical experience with dying patients should have schooled him and made him sensitive to the varied attitudes of people as they draw nearer to death. The physician acts wisely and truthfully if, with the greatest reverence, he helps the patient to 'mature' his death as suggested by Rainer Maria Rilke's prayer, 'O Lord, give everyone his own death, the dying which proceeds from that life in which we had love, meaning and anguish ... for this makes dying strange and difficult that it is not our death; it is one which takes us at last because we have not matured our own.' [5]

---

[5] Cf.: R.J. Bulger, 'Doctors and Dying,' *Archives of Internal Medicine*, 112 (September, 1963), 81-86.

J

At this crucial point, the doctor's initiative confines itself to helping the patient to arrive at the truthfulness of his own life as directly as possible. It is not only through words but through his whole deportment that the doctor leads his patient to the realization of the seriousness of his situation. Having established with him a relationship of mutual trust, he knows intuitively the extent to which the patient wishes to be informed. Whether the patient asks directly in so many words or indirectly through his probing comments to the physician, he has always the right to be apprized of his situation in so far as this constitutes a portion of that truth required for the most decisive response.

An experienced physician writes, 'The truth of the real situation is usually withheld from the patient, and this misrepresentation about his condition involves him in a game of deception.... If there is any honour left in his life and any dignity in his dying, should not the patient have the right to make a choice for himself about his destiny on the basis of truth?' [6]

While modern man has learned that attitudes towards sex tend to become healthier when brought into the open for discussion, the subject of death remains a taboo for many doctors, even in cases where the patient has outgrown the infantilism of taboos. 'Somehow many of us have come to believe that we have a right to lie to patients on the assumption that we are protecting them from the cruelties and realities of life and death. This is the first step in the destruction of an honest relationship with the patient.' [7] A nun who had served in the hospital nursing services for thirty years and whom I visited when she was in the terminal stages of carcinoma said to me, 'The greatest insult to my intelligence and to my faith is the doctor's effort to lie to me and the cowardice of my superior who complies with his order

[6] John C. Conley, 'Rights of the Dying Patient,' (editorial), *Archives of Otolaryngology*, 90 (October, 1969), 405.
[7] W.H. Baltzell, 'The Dying Patient — When the Focus Must be Changed,' *Archives of Internal Medicine*, 127 (January, 1971), 108.

to do the same.' Often doctors are the culprits 'who suggest to the family that they conceal the truth from the patient' although the latter is prepared to hear the truth. 'Why do we do this destructive thing? The integrity of the family structure is weakened at a time when it should be strong, strong enough to give tenderness to the patient and comfort to the survivors. It is not possible to be tender to someone whose eye you cannot meet.' [8]

The doctor has a professional obligation to inform the patient of his situation as fully as the patient reasonably wishes to know it. Of course, there should always be a liberal admixture of hope and sympathy. While expressing his professional opinion, the doctor will indicate that it represents no more than an estimate of probabilities and that no doctor's judgment can be considered infallible. He will refrain from informing the patient suddenly, meting out all the facts at once. Instead, he will reveal the gravity of the situation step by step according to the patient's ability to cope with it and, of course, according to the time left for such a preparation.

In many instances, the physician relies on the members of the family to impart such information to the dying. He usually presents them first with the full picture of the patient's condition, explaining the medical angles adequately, but he would be remiss in his duty were he to overlook the human aspects related to the task of sharing such knowledge.

If the patient indicates clearly, explicitly or implicitly, that he does not want the whole truth, this wish must be respected as much as possible. The wisest course of action for the physician is to allow the patient an opportunity to exercise his choice about learning the reality of his condition. I am not implying that the doctor simply await the patient's request for the facts; rather, he will speak to the patient in such a way as to invite acceptance or refusal of fuller information depending on his readiness at that

---

[8] *Ibid.*

particular time.[9] 'Some preliminary studies suggest that, while most physicians do not favour telling their patients about impending death, most patients desire to be told frankly though gently about their condition as they approach death. When they do receive such information, they usually demonstrate a high capacity for handling the communication either in an open manner or in defensive ways that protect them from trauma.'[10] A number of experiments seem to indicate that this is true even with respect to children.[11]

Any actual deception is to be excluded in favour of a doctor-patient relationship which assures the magnanimous fulfilment of the medical vocation. It would surely be a help towards this if all doctors would observe this principle: 'Never, under any condition, should patients be told untruths. This is the surest way to destroy the mutual trust and respect which in the end may prove to be the most important therapeutic asset the physician possesses.'[12]

Often enough the patient is reluctant to see a priest because, to his mind or to that of the family, the clergyman's appearance on the scene presages the beginning of the end to life's journey. But even if the priest is available and the patient accepts him, the doctor is not absolved from concern relative to his patient's emotional and spiritual problems. In the years of my medical military service, I experienced often how very different was the situation of my meeting the dying soldier as a priest only or as one also who could assist him in his physical distress and try to save his life. The dying man was not receiving

---

[9] Cf.: C.K. Aldrich, 'The Dying Patient's Grief,' *Journal of the American Medical Association,* 184 (May, 1963), 331.

[10] A.L. Knutson, 'Cultural Beliefs on Life and Death,' in *The Dying Patient,* ed. Orville G. Brim *et al.* (New York: Russell Sage Foundation, 1970), p. 60. There is extensive documentation to this study.

[11] J. Vernick and M. Karon, 'Who's Afraid of Death in a Leukemia Ward?' *American Journal of Diseases of Children,* 109 (May, 1965), 393-397.

[12] P.S. Rhoads, 'Management of the Patient with Terminal Illness,' *Journal of the American Medical Association,* 192 (May, 1965), 78.

the same message; the psychological resonance, the readiness and gratitude differed markedly.

The word of the physician is often an indispensable testimony for the patient. The mere fact that his physician is aware of the spiritual dimension of his plight is immensely important to him. Truthful information is to be seen in this light. It has nothing to do with the loveless flinging of truth in the face of an anxious patient. Rather, it is an authentic way of befriending him as he searches for the ultimate truth of his life. Such a gesture on the part of his doctor will intimate the presence of the Divine Physician whose Truth is communicated with the healing power of love.

4. The physician's rôle following the patient's death

With the death of the patient, the professional rôle of the physician has not yet terminated. It belongs to his task and vocation to assist the members of the family beyond the hour of death through manifestations of sympathy and understanding, but above all, through that encouragement which helps them overcome emotional imbalance. The more he holds the trust of the family, the more irreplaceable will be his moral support after the patient's death.

C. The moment of death

Determining the exact time of death has been a major concern of man throughout history. With the development of resuscitation procedures used early after the usual signs of death, the whole question of the 'moment of death' reached a new phase. It took the first heart transplant, however, truly to revolutionize the traditional approach. The mystique of the heart is now gone; the heart is an important pump which can be replaced by that of a just-deceased person or, possibly in the future, by a plastic heart. The general public suddenly came to realize that the moment of death cannot be determined by the function of the heart. Not only is the biological basis of death being redefined but many other new insights are coming to the fore concerning the substratum of the life history of human beings.

1. Medical breakthroughs

When the problem of resuscitation was first posed, Pius XII declared in one of his discourses: 'It is in the physician's domain . . . to give a clear and precise definition of "death" and of the "moment of death" of a patient who dies without regaining consciousness. In such a case, one can refer to the usual concept of separation . . . of the soul from the body; but on the practical level, one needs to be mindful of the connotation of the terms "body" and "separation". . . . As to the pronouncement of death in certain particular cases, the answer cannot be inferred from religious and moral principles, and consequently, it is an aspect lying outside the competence of the Church.' [13]

Medical science the world over confronted the problem of defining the moment of death with new thoroughness after the first heart transplant. It seems that these new surgical advances benefited humanity not so much by the prolongation of the life of a few individuals as by the attainment of new insights relative to the moment of death and the furtherance of knowledge about human existence.

2. Brain death = human death

Even prior to the first heart transplant, science knew of the unique importance of the cerebral cortex as the centre of consciousness and voluntary action. Only in the new context, however, has a general consensus been reached that brain death is the end of the earthly history of a human person. 'The brain only gives man his reality; where it has disappeared, man no longer is. Such is also the opinion expressed by the leading national and international medical authorities.' [14] The principle

---

[13] Pius XII, *Acta Apostolicae Sedis,* 45 (November, 1957), 1027-1033.
[14] M. Goulon and P. Babinet, 'Le coma dépassé,' *Cahiers Laennec,* (September, 1970), 18.

that brain death is synonymous with the death of the patient
has found universal agreement. The consequences are most
relevant: 'After brain death, the surgeon has the moral obligation to stop all artificial methods of sustaining life by
respirators.' [15]

3. Biological life prolonged

Determination of the moment of death through the equation
of man's death with brain death is more than a scientific question.
Without a holistic vision of man, how could anyone arrive at
the conviction that no human life is given without the substratum
essential for typically personal activity? After brain death, important human organs such as the heart, lungs, kidneys and liver
can be kept functioning by artificial means. In spite of the fact
that organic life continues to exist, without the substratum of
consciousness, freedom and affectivity, that is, without the centre
that organizes and gives human meaning to this organic life, there
can no longer be question of the history of a human person.

Today, the question is extended further by accumulated
biological knowledge and correlative reflection. While the primitive brain provides the regulation centres for the dynamic order
of man's whole biological organism, the cerebral cortex is the
decisive organ which makes possible the various forms of
spiritual expression. With the destruction of the cerebral cortex,
the material substratum for any spiritual activity is destroyed;
man no longer has the possibility of realizing his personality in
freedom and his human history comes to an end. The loss of
those cortical centres absolutely necessary for consciousness and
typically human expression makes it highly probable that human
personal life has run its course even if other functions of the
primitive brain can be maintained for the preservation of organic
life in its biological organization.[16] Here, however, we are faced

---

[15] Lyman A. Brewer, 'De Humanitate,' *The American Journal of
Surgery*, 118 (August, 1969), 136.
[16] W. Ruff, 'Individualität und Personalität in embryonalen Werden,'
Theologie und Philosophie, op. cit., 45 (1970), p. 47.

with a problem calling for further research and discussion. The consequences are most relevant not only for heart transplants but, among other things, for the determination of the point beyond which mere prolongation of the biological life of man would be senseless.

4. Death redefined

With respect to the practical determination of the moment of death, particularly for the ablation of organs needed in transplants, medicine is choosing the safest course. It insists on total brain death, that is, the destruction of those parts of the brain (primitive brain) which regulate the biological functioning of the body. 'We are sure that the linear tracing (not a "flat" nor a "coma" EEG reading) and the absence of spontaneous respiration indicate that the central nervous system has ceased functioning from head to foot, from the cortex down; to our knowledge, no one has ever seen such a subject recover any cerebral function whatsoever.' [17]

An authoritative formulation of criteria for death in the case of prospective organ donors was proposed by a distinguished interdisciplinary group of surgeons, jurists and clergymen who met in London in 1966 for the purpose of discussing the ethical considerations of the new surgical procedures. Basically, the five criteria were: complete dilation of the pupils with no reflex response to light; complete absence of muscle and tendon reflexes to usual stimuli; complete absence of spontaneous respiration after the mechanical respirator has been stopped for five minutes; constantly dropping blood pressure in spite of massive doses of vasopressor drugs and a flat EEG tracing for several minutes. Complete cessation of heartbeat was no longer considered evidence of death.[18]

---

[17] H. Fishgold, 'Electroencephalographe et signes de la mort,' *Cahiers Laennec*, (September, 1970), 50.

[18] Paul S. Rhoads, 'Moral Considerations in Prolongation of Life,' *Journal of the South Carolina Medical Association*, (October, 1968), 422-423.

In the wake of the Capetown furore, a Harvard University team later studied carefully the entire 'organ transplant' problem, and in suggesting its own norms, dismissed the 'drop in blood pressure' posited by the Alexandre team and added strictures to the other criteria. In summary, the Harvard committee 'stated that in order for brain death to be designated, the subject should be in deep and irreversible coma; manifest a total unawareness to external painful stimuli; have no spontaneous muscular movements or elicitable reflexes; have pupils fixed, dilated, and unresponsive to light; and have an isolectric EEG, with the foregoing characteristics having been maintained over a period of twenty-four hours.' [19]

It is somewhat surprising that medical authorities and other participants in the interdisciplinary dialogue on heart transplant now demand a much higher degree of certitude about death than they did previously when the donor's organs would not have rendered any life-saving service to others. However, the discussions lead also to some practical results bearing on that moment at which further efforts at prolonging life can or should be stopped. The criteria required for irreversible brain death are extremely severe. There is a general trend towards the conviction that brain death should be ascertained by a team other than the transplant team.

For potential transplants where organs are removed from deceased persons, it is absolutely necessary that the organs should not have lost their biological life. Thus, for some there remains a doubt — though a slight theoretical doubt — as to whether the total death of man has occurred with brain death, although it is agreed that the unalterable process of dying is assured. They therefore come to the conclusion that, in this case, the excision of the organ could still have the character of homicide or of anticipating total death. Even on this presupposition, however,

---

[19] Beecher, Henry K. *et al.*, 'A definition of irreversible coma. Report of the Ad Hoc Committee of the Harvard Medical School to Examine the Definition of Brain Death,' *Journal of the American Medical Association*, 205 (August 5, 1968), 337-340.

traditional interpretations of the command 'Thou shalt not kill' would most probably allow this slight anticipation of the moment of total death where the whole process of dying is irrevocable because no new cause of death would be introduced; there is simply a speeding of the final process of decay. At any rate, the history of human existence in the sense of truly personal life would not be shortened.[20] Personally, I feel that the arguments for the equation of the total death of the person with brain death are fully valid.

5. Mechanical support for transferable organs

Now that it is possible to keep organs alive for hours, days, and even longer by chemical and mechanical means, the question arises: is it not against the dignity of the human person to maintain organs and tissues artificially after brain death in order to have them available for transplants later? There is no doubt that these procedures constitute manipulation, but they affect only parts of a human body which do not have the status of a living person. The response to the question flows from our understanding of human nature. During one's lifetime, health and sometimes life itself are exposed to risks in the service of one's neighbour. Is it not in keeping with the dialogical nature of man to have one's organs, even after death, continue a life dedicated to the service of others in the form of a transplanted organ?[21]

Of course, with respect to the freedom with which one can dispose of one's own organs after death, juridical problems relative to their use and the rights of the family have to be resolved, but from a moral point of view, if our earthly life has rightfully come to its end, not the slightest objection can be set forth against the life-saving use of our organs in the body of some other person.

---

[20] Cf.. H. Pompey, 'Gehirntod und totaler Tod,' *Münchener Medizinische Wochenschrift,* 13 (1969), 736-741.

[21] Cf.: B. Casper, 'Der Tod als menschliches Phänomen,' *Arzt und Christ,* 15 (1969), 160.

D. *Organ transplant*

Up to this point, we have treated the transplantation of organs in relation to the moment of death only. Further light will be shed on it in our discussion of the prolongation of life. Some additional points beyond these fundamental questions remain to be considered.

Kidney transplants which seemed to be either impossible or an unreasonable risk a few years ago have now a high rate of success, saving hundreds of lives yearly. Originally, the immunologic problems seemed insuperable: only the kidneys of the mother or of an identical twin could be life-saving. Today the surgical feats of transplantation extend to many other organs. Transplanting corneas from the eyes of recently deceased persons gives back sight to countless people, and there is now a promising prospect for the transplant of lungs and liver. It is evident, then, that the transplantation of organs from a living person (for example, of kidneys) will no longer be justified if the same result can be obtained through cadaver organs. However, there might still be cases in which only an immediate kidney transplant using the organ of a living person could save a precious life. The sacrifice of a kidney whose loss would not endanger one's life and activity is to be measured by the great command of love. It is unreasonable to condemn this action as an intrinsically evil self-mutilation since the total meaning of the act determines its morality.

Each case has to be resolved in view of the good of both persons, the recipient and the donor, in a freely responsible decision to bestow and to accept such a telling sign of love.[22] Enlightened responsibility obliges the prospective donor to weigh carefully the giving of one of his organs so that he does not harm himself beyond proper limits and does not fundamentally imperil his obligations towards other persons. If the

---

[22] Cf.: A. Regan, C.Ss.R., 'Man's Administration of His Bodily Life and Members, the Principle of Totality and Organic Transplants Between Humans,' *Studia Moralia,* V (Rome, 1967), 179-200.

recipient is conscious, he must not accept an offer which cannot be made wisely. It is the doctor's duty to inform the persons involved to the best of his knowledge about the risks incurred and to help them arrive at a prudent decision.

An important criterion for organ transplant relates to the possible consequences of such surgery with respect to one's identity and the development of personal freedom. Years ago Pius XII stated that the transfer of an animal sex gland would have to be rejected as immoral because of the great disturbance of freedom which would be likely to follow.[23] The integrity of personal life and of a person's identity prevail over prolonging life or any other possible advantage accruing from a transplant. With respect to heart or lung transplants, there is no reason to fear a dangerous modification of the personality. A transplanted heart 'is less apt to injure the spiritual personality of the recipient than are certain currently accepted psychiatric and neurosurgical techniques.'[24]

E. *The prolongation of life*

Since the physician's task has always been to engage in battle against death, the problem of prolonging life cannot be looked upon as new. However, the situation has changed so much that totally new aspects have emerged.

1. *The newness of the problem*

In pre-scientific times, newborn babies who could never come to a proper use of human freedom or even to full consciousness were irrevocably destined to die. At the present stage of medical progress, some of these lives can be prolonged for

---

[23] Pius XII, *A.A.S.*, 48 (May 14, 1956), 460. See also my book: *The Law of Christ*, III, pp. 241-243; 692-693.

[24] Charles Dubost, 'Scientific and Ethical Problems in Organ Transplantation,' *The Annals of Thoracic Surgery*, 8 (August, 1969), 102.

several months and in other cases for several years. Even more
astonishing strides can be expected with respect to the prolongation of life for the aged. Where the traditional medical practice
of a few decades ago would have pronounced 'death' as a *fait
accompli*, today resuscitation procedures give many a new lease
of life. Organ transplant represents another medical advance
which can save, or at least extend, a life formerly doomed to
death.

While in earlier times most people died in the midst of their
families, statistics in the United States disclose that well over
eighty per cent now die in hospitals, where all means of prolonging
life are close at hand. Very often these people end their days
in a state of psychological isolation and estrangement, with tubes
in every orifice and needles in their veins while waiting to draw
their last breath. 'Heroic efforts are made to keep them breathing
as long as possible even by using a heart-lung machine if one is
available.' In many cases, these techniques 'may insure prolongation of vital signs but certainly cannot be called "prolongation
of life".' [25] 'We have all seen instances of an *organism* maintained
alive after all hope for the person's returning to life was
irretrievably gone.' [26]

In view of the meticulous concern manifested by the
strictures imposed on the medical profession in the matter of
determining human death, we can now question the consistency
of those physicians who hold to their very dubious 'liberal' stance
with regard to the deliberate ending of fetal life without a similar
effort to determine safely and certainly the *beginning* of human
life. In many countries there is monstrous disproportion between
disregard or even contempt for human life in its promising
beginning and the great concern for prolonging death, even
by maintaining biological functions through artificial means in a
'brain dead' body.

---

[25] Ch. U. Letourneau, 'Dying with Dignity,' *Hospital Management*,
(June, 1970), 30.
[26] P.F. Regan, 'The Dying Patient,' *op. cit.* p. 83.

2. *The ethical right to die in dignity*

Many hard questions arise from the new insights and the new power of medicine. One which is being increasingly raised among doctors, nurses and the population at large is the right of the person to die with dignity and grace. This has nothing to do with the problem of euthanasia which will be treated later. The problem is posed in an anguished way if resuscitation is attempted when it is most probable that the major cortical centres are irreparably damaged or destroyed. The question is: should a person who has always manifested maturity and wisdom now be artificially kept 'alive' for months or years in a fully unconscious state or in one of obvious mental absence or grave disturbance? This represents only one of the extreme cases where modern techniques reverse the course of 'nature.' It is no wonder that we hear the clamour of more and more voices asserting that it is immoral to prolong life artificially when, in particular situations, this means only prolonging suffering, the agony or the act of death. Pius XII long ago spoke in an approving tone about families who bring pressure to bear upon the attending physician 'to remove the respirators so as to allow the patient, already virtually dead, to depart in peace.' [27] Medical progress must not deny a person his ethical right to die in human dignity.[28]

3. *Criteria for prolonging life*

Among theologians, there is probably no one who has stated the problem of criteria so strongly as Thielicke. 'If we speak about the duty of the doctor to preserve life, then not biological life as such is meant but *human* life. In order to characterize the

---

[27] Pius XII, Discourse to Doctors (November 24, 1957), *A.A.S.*, 49 (1957), 1029.
[28] Cf.: W.J. Boone, 'Religion and Medicine,' *Journal of the Medical Society of New Jersey*, 65 (1968), 637.
Cf.: See also, A. Gütgemann, 'Uber arztliche Verantwortung in der Chirurgie,' *Münchener Medizinische Wochenschrift*, 17 (1967), 14.

life of man, other criteria are needed than those of the electro-
cardiograph and the electroencephalograph.' [29]

The first tentative criterion is an educated estimate of the
hoped-for prolongation of life and the amount of suffering and
disenchantment which this prolonged life may cause to the
patient and his family. Why prolong life if it is only to bring
greater disillusionment and temptation? In this respect the
economic factor must surely never play the main *rôle*, but it can
truly become a matter of justice, charity and human concern.
Consider a father who has worked hard and lived frugally all
his life in order to assure a good education for his children;
what tremendous suffering it must be for him to see the slight
prolongation of his now hopeless life drain all his savings and
resources needed for the children's future. Positively formulated,
this criterion indicates that if there is a well-grounded or even
faint hope of prolonging life in such a way that a reasonably
happy and significant existence can be anticipated for a short or
longer period of time, then every possible means at our disposal
should be used.[30]

What 'possible means' signifies has to be determined from a
medical point of view, and by evaluating all human aspects and
duties calling for consideration. The doctor must not allow the
family to seduce him to the point of using the most expensive
procedures for the sole purpose of appeasing them when there
is practically no hope that it would be of any avail to the patient.
An expensive treatment for a life already doomed may constitute
a grave injustice towards the members of the patient's family.
Often the heavy financial burden is incurred by the family
solely through fear for their reputation. The attending physician
would be acting irresponsibly were he to yield to family
pressures in such a case.

Kautzky gives as the principal criterion a meaningful
development of human freedom. 'Since human life is the condi-

---

[29] H. Thielicke, 'Ethische Fragen der modernen Medizin,' *Archiv für
klinische Chirurgie*, 321 (1968), 13.
[30] Cf.: P.S. Rhoads, 'Moral Considerations,' *op. cit.*, 428.

tion for the realization of human freedom, it should be prolonged with all appropriate and reasonable means insofar as prolongation according to a competent estimate can serve this goal.' [31] I agree with the criterion which makes fundamental the promotion of human freedom only if an individualistic misinterpretation of freedom is excluded. Loving care for the sick members of one's family or even for strangers, for bodily and mentally disabled children and the like, represents a culmination of the history of genuine freedom on the part of those who dedicate themselves freely and generously out of respect for human dignity.

At this point, however, we are considering the particular question of prolonging a life artificially where the patient will never again come to any reasonable use of his own freedom. This is where I agree with the physician: 'Not each prolongation of life is a gain of freedom. It can be defeated by total lack of consciousness, grave defects and suffering of all kinds. Therefore pain and excruciating suffering must be conquered by medication even if this would cause an earlier death.' [32] However, in the case of those who are absolutely willing and able to accept a reasonable amount of suffering, sedatives must not be used to the extent that the patients' freedom would be eliminated by their being kept in a continual state of unconsciousness.

Realization of significant liberty for man in the total history of human freedom and redemption absolutely precludes the impersonal criterion of 'usefulness' which branded the cruelties of Hitler. A society which predicates the saving of life in terms of economic utility only and the doctors entrapped in this mode of thinking have already betrayed the history of freedom. Therefore caution should be exercised in the use of an expression such as 'useful life' when one means something as totally different as 'meaningful life.' The three hours of Christ on the cross were the most significant moments of human history.

If we take freedom as the main criterion, then it is obvious that the free choice of the patient must be in the foreground of

---

[31] R. Kautzky, 'Der Arzt,' *Arzt und Christ,* 15 (1969), 138.
[32] *Ibid.*

all considerations. Is he well-prepared for death and does he
express an objective and calmly acquired decision that his life
should not be prolonged artificially through extraordinary interventions? If so, this desire is to be respected even if one of the
chief motives of the dying person is to avoid added burdens and
harmful debts for his family. The predominant motive here is
not one of utility but an expression of loving concern and
responsibility. I repeat that I am not referring here to
euthanasia but only to cases where artificial measures for the
prolongation of life could or should be stopped, especially when
there is no hope whatsoever that health can be regained. I wish
to emphasize the need for a sharp distinction between cases
where there is a *real* chance of serving human life compared to
other cases where physicians would be merely interfering with
death or sustaining artificially the process of death.

Traditional moral theology distinguished between ordinary
and extraordinary means of saving life. Earlier moralists knew
nothing of the present staggering possibilities of prolonging the
process of death when a person is virtually dead. In my opinion,
neither with ordinary nor with extraordinary means should
death be dramatized and prolonged. Otherwise, in the near future,
heart-lung machines would have to be used in all cases since
they would be 'ordinary means' in wealthy countries. But where
there is truly a prolongation of human life, the principles formulated earlier by Pius XII maintain their full validity: 'Natural
reason and Christian morals say that man has the right and the
duty in case of serious illness to take the necessary treatment for
the preservation of life and health. This duty that he has towards
himself, towards God, towards the human community, and in
most cases towards certain determined persons, derives from
well-ordered charity, from submission to the Creator, from social
justice, as well as from devotion towards his family.

'But normally, one is held to use only ordinary means —
according to circumstances of persons, places, times, and
culture — that is to say, means that do not involve any grave
burden for oneself or another. A more strict obligation would
be too burdensome for most men and would render the attain-

K

ment of the higher, more important good too difficult. Life, death,
all temporal activities are in fact subordinated to spiritual ends.
On the other hand, one is not forbidden to take more than
strictly necessary steps to preserve life and health, as long as one
does not fail in some more serious duty.' [33]

F. Euthanasia

The word euthanasia is of Greek origin and originally
signified a good and honourable death. In medical language, it
has always expressed the kind assistance which the physician
gave to the dying patient in order to alleviate his suffering, to
diminish pain and anguish. It is only in the course of the
twentieth century that the friendly word came to mean the
direct and painless killing of a patient who, lacking the prospect
of recovering health, might want this kind of immediate death.
Binding and Hoche proposed, under this name of euthanasia, the
premeditated and large-scale planned extermination of socially
and economically 'unfit' persons, especially the mentally ill, and
the crippled who might impede economic progress.[34] This is the
euthanasia practised by Hitler; besides millions of 'undesired'
Jews, he executed hundreds of thousands of mentally or physically handicapped persons of his own nation.

The present discussion of euthanasia reported in the
professional literature reveals that everyone is most eager to
dissociate his proposals from the mass crimes of Hitler; however,
expressions like 'useless life' constantly recur and for any number
of justifications.

1. Distinctions needed

Physicians usually distinguish between negative and positive
euthanasia. By negative euthanasia is meant the planned omission

---

[33] Pius XII, A.A.S., 49 (1957), 1031-1032.
[34] Karl Binding and Alfred Hoche, Die Freigabe der Vernichtung
lebensunwerten Lebens (Leipzig, 1920).

of treatments that would probably prolong life; *positive euthanasia* refers to the proposed institution of 'therapies' designed to promote death sooner than would be expected otherwise.[35] Positive euthanasia is sometimes called 'mercy killing,' although of late physicians cringe from any association with these words because of their shocking connotation. Indeed, the direct intention of positive euthanasia *is* to put an end to the patient's life. The chief motive advanced is that of 'compassion,' at least in the arguments used. In medical discussions, positive euthanasia is considered as object of deliberation only in so far as the patient has unambiguously expressed the desire that the doctor should, in an 'act of mercy,' positively cooperate in hastening death.

2. *Negative euthanasia: problems*

The expression 'negative euthanasia' can have a variety of meanings. From a moral point of view, a number of distinctions need to be made.

The numerous Christian Scientists who believe that nature ought always to be permitted to take its course, the Witnesses of Jehovah who consider even a blood transfusion immoral, a Catholic doctor who decides to let a pregnant woman die since he was taught that the only life-saving action open to him would be an immoral 'direct' abortion (an extremely rare case) — all, on the practical level, refuse a treatment which doctors at large consider normal for preserving life. However, none of these would consider as positive or negative euthanasia their decision to allow death to come to the patient, nor would the expression 'negative euthanasia' usually be applied to these cases since the motive never purported incidental death. The withholding of life-saving procedures involves a very serious decision for the doctor or for the family, but it is arrived at only because of the fear that the prolongation of life would entail recourse to immoral means. Negative euthanasia applies only to cases in

---

[35] R.H. Williams, 'Our Role,' *Archives of Internal Medicine, op. cit.,* p. 229.

which practically all hope of saving the life of the patient has disappeared and where the direct question is one of prolonging the terminal illness or ending it sooner through discontinuance of therapy.

In some non-Catholic circles there would be no hesitation in labelling as negative euthanasia the decision not to prolong life according to the principles enunciated by Pius XII in 1957. However, for the sake of clarity, it has to be said that there is a real difference in whether the direct objective (as in the Pius XII doctrine) is to dispense with *extraordinary* means or to stop treatments altogether in order to allow the patient to die (negative euthanasia with a number of nuances). In the Catholic tradition, there is no reluctance to approve of treatments whose direct purpose is the suppression of undesirable pain and anxiety — even though a shortening of the terminal illness might be foreseen. It is another thing, however, to stop treatments specifically in order to hasten death. Also different is the stopping only of those treatments which instead of really prolonging life, only prolong the process of death.

I trust that the non-Catholic reader will not consider these as hairsplitting distinctions. Protestant theologians often make the same distinctions, although generally with lesser emphasis. I quote one of the best known Protestant ethicists: 'Of course it does make a great difference whether I accept an evil or a questionable result only as a by-product of my therapeutic intention or seek it directly as a good in itself. The decisive ethical difference between goal and by-product has been familiar to us at all times in other medical contexts. It plays a *rôle* in the question of euthanasia: I may accept death or the anticipation of death as a possible risk inherent in other therapeutic or analgesic treatments.' [36] There are quite a few surgical interventions with a fifty per cent probability of success. Up to now, medical ethics has not objected when these procedures were the only alternatives to a few months of a most miserable life. On

---

[36] H. Thielicke, 'Ethische Fragen,' *op. cit.,* p. 18.

this basis, the first transplants were justified. They have nothing
to do with the problem of euthanasia.

Taken in the strictest sense, negative euthanasia *by direct
intention* approaches the shortening of agony or even of a fatal
disease (which could last months) through planned withdrawal
or omission of life-prolonging treatment. Although normally
such treatments are in the category traditionally considered
'extraordinary,' this distinction does not constitute their rationale.
The straightforward intention is: not to prolong that suffering
which is considered opposed to the idea of dying in dignity and
peace. It is looked upon as the response to a new situation
caused by the unusual progress of medicine.

What are the physician's thoughts on negative euthanasia?
Williams reports on a survey pertaining to a systematic polling
of opinion on antifertility measures, abortion, euthanasia and
transplants. The respondents were chairmen of medical depart-
ments in the United States' schools of medicine and members of
the Association of American Physicians. Of the three hundred
and forty-four questionnaires sent out, three hundred and thirty-
three were returned (a ninety-seven per cent response). Of
the three hundred and thirty-three respondents, eighty-seven
per cent voted in favour of negative euthanasia, but only eighty
per cent indicated that they did practise negative euthanasia,
Protestants the most (eighty-eight per cent) and Catholic doctors
the least (sixty-two per cent).[37]

The ethical question remains: is the premeditated omission
of treatments with the direct intention not to prolong the
process of dying morally good or not? In my opinion,
we have to be most careful not to rush in with a negative judgment, if the decision rests strictly within the criteria posited
earlier with respect to the prolongation of life.[38] However,
negative euthanasia is to be formally rejected if the concept is
unduly enlarged and if considerations of bare utility enter into
the picture. There are tendencies in some discussions not only

---

[37] R.H. Williams, 'Our Role,' *op. cit.*, p. 230.
[38] See section E of this chapter.

to allow the patient to die in dignity but, through the withholding of treatment, to intend directly the elimination, in an unostentatious way, of those who most probably would have a long sickly life or be unable to insert themselves into the economic process. Therefore, it is imperative that the medical profession take a strong anti-utility stand in view of the increasing number of those favouring positive euthanasia and others introducing a falsified defintion of negative euthanasia.

3. 'No' to positive euthanasia

In the inquiry of Williams, which was mentioned above, only very few Protestant and Jewish doctors and not a single Catholic doctor voted in favour of positive euthanasia, but up to thirty-eight per cent of the others favoured it. The last years have recorded heated discussions on the problem in England.[39] As in many other important ethical questions, it could well be that the decisions in England will have a far-reaching impact on similar decisions in other countries. In the House of Lords, forty per cent of the membership voted for a bill that would have legalized positive euthanasia although only under well-determined conditions, such as a spontaneous and free decision of the patient and a thirty day interim between statement of interest and execution.

That we have to speak out firmly against the idea of positive euthanasia there should be no doubt; but, in the long run, success can be hoped for only if we override a utilitarian philosophy and strengthen the respect for each person, and if humanity sees the beneficial meaning of the commandment 'Thou shalt not kill' in all sectors of life. Physicians should be the first to mobilize public opinion because they can fully visualize how their whole relationship to the sick would be changed if positive euthanasia became institutionalized.

Which are the valid and convincing arguments and motives to be marshalled in this situation? In earlier times, the general

---

[39] 'Killing of Patients,' *British Medical Journal,* 5 (April, 1969), 4-5.

argument, 'You may not choose when to fall into the arms of God who alone is Lord over life and death' seemed sufficient. Today, however, it is not as simple as that because Christian Scientists and the Witnesses of Jehovah invoke this argument equally in proscribing blood transfusions. Neither can our argument be the old slogan, 'Let nature run its own course,' for the problem of artificial prolongation of life and of the strictly medical discussion of negative euthanasia arises chiefly from the fact that modern medicine controls the course of nature. Artificial respiration and resuscitation are most striking examples of medicine's not allowing nature to run havoc with life. I think that, for the believer, the strongest argument against euthanasia is in the perspective of *freedom*. The so-called 'free choice' of death, that is, forcing death to take us at the moment and under the conditions we stipulate, would 'not increase but diminish the fullness of the free acceptance of death, which is the course we have chosen. To exercise freedom's choice in life according to our own power, and in death according to our powerlessness, is the most truthful admission of our creaturely human existence in these two realities. This choice is the only acceptable foundation on which we have to build day after day.' [40]

From a more practical point of view, many rightly insist on the wedge reaction. If euthanasia were legalized and brought into today's philosophy of man's economic utility, who would finally make the decision? The persons *'mercifully'* to be killed might well, because of their condition, be unfit to make a rational decision based on unwavering conviction. 'Quite possibly they might be influenced by worry about the trouble they are causing their family, and, as Lady Summerskill said, "undoubtedly there would be somebody to remind the invalid of his newly acquired powers over his own disposal." Is a sense of guilt at being alive to be added to a feeling of resignation — let alone regret — at dying?' [41]

---

[40] R. Kautzky, 'Der Arzt,' *op. cit.*, p. 138.
[41] 'Killing of Patients,' *op. cit.*, p. 4.

Already, we know of the increasing number of suicides among the aged; in Scandinavia, for instance, society's attitude informs the elderly that they have passed the point of 'usefulness.' While the discussions on negative euthanasia centre mainly on some tragic but marginal cases, do the discussions on positive euthanasia unmask the horrifying situation of a humanity that has lost its understanding of life and death? They are unquestionably marked by that attitude which led Hitler to distinguish between 'fit' and 'unfit' life.

We have to be fully aware of the difficulty of providing convincing motives for those who do not believe in the death-passion-resurrection of Christ, and who have also been unable to grasp the full value of suffering and of selfless service to suffering mankind. So we have here a touchstone of the medical ethos and ethics at large.

G. *Merciless killing*

Between 1949 and 1967, there were 16,395,616 abortions registered in Japan. The full responsibility does not lie with Japan. Political pressure was exerted by foreign powers to stem population growth through abortion. North American sociologists and psychologists crusaded and moulded the opinion of the Japanese public and of their legislators. Guilt is imputable also to those nations who have denied living space to Orientals. Australia, for instance, with only thirteen million inhabitants, refuses immigration to the yellow race. To a considerable extent, the fault lies also with those who refused to distinguish between contraception and abortion and therefore could not exert their moral influence against abortion. This massive flood of killing by abortion has now reached the United States. In New York City alone, in the first year of legalized abortion, 164,000 pre-natal lives were violently ended.

The Second World War killed no less than twenty million men. Over the past decade highway fatalities in Europe have ranged from 85,000 to 100,000 annually. In the United States the number is over 50,000. This means that during the last ten years, in the more highly industrialized countries — which, out of respect for life have taken decisive steps to eliminate capital punishment — more than two million people have been killed on the roads by reckless or negligent drivers.

In comparison with these statistics, the most discussed risk of constructive medical interventions does not seem to weigh too heavily. Nevertheless, the medical profession has to cast all its decisions and discussions in this context: it cannot be indifferent to mass killings of any kind if it wants to preserve and to deepen its life-saving ethos in this age. Individually and collectively through their organizations, physicians must take an active *rôle* in efforts to build a worldwide social philosophy of humaneness, of peace among men, and of individual care for the health and lives of others.

Chapter 8

THE HEALTH OF MAN

The ethics of the medical profession pivot on its answers to three questions which have already been discussed, namely, what is the nature of man? (chapter 5), what is human life? (chapter 6), what is death? (chapter 7), and a fourth question which I purpose to treat here, what is human health?

Our holistic approach to life, death and health gives this chapter its direction and its particular interest. The discussion cannot be restricted to the physician-patient relationship but properly encompasses the whole health-illness continuum. The range of issues to be covered is by no means exhaustive; special attention will be given to: psychopathology and therapy; the general problems of health care with an eye to prophylaxis and the duty befalling everyone and every community to create humane living conditions with a view to optimal human health; current ethical issues in the medical profession and experimentation with human subjects.

A. *The concept of health and illness*

The concepts of health care are as varied and numerous as those of man's nature, life and death. Though different, these notions of health usually do not contradict one another; they are even complementary when they are neither closed nor made absolute.

1. Health: more than physical fitness

Health, like human nature, has an altogether social finality. As a group endowment, it attests to the cooperation and interdependence of people in the fields of nourishment, housing, prenatal and child care, education, care of society's dependent members, and the shaping of the physical-psychological environment. As a social responsibility, it appeals to everyone's ability and generosity to serve the fundamental social groups of family and community. In the past, whenever failing health rendered people incapable of discharging the duties expected of them by their family or society, the doctor was summoned. This has always been true, but the emergence of new social rôles for the doctor, for example, as school physician or industrial doctor, and the physicians' dependence on health insurances have wrought changes in the medical man's Gestalt.

In a utilitarian age, there is a mounting temptation to define health chiefly or simply in terms of capacity for work, physical fitness or the ability of a man to perform a certain function, whatever it may be.[1] The physician may be seduced to the point of overlooking the patient's inability to fulfil adequately his other rôles of spouse, parent or citizen. The emphasis on physical fitness becomes exceptionally dangerous when rooted in a public opinion geared primarily to utility. An authoritarian state can then capitalize on this ideology, classify its citizens according to their efficiency and utility to the state, and even try to eliminate those who fail to serve its economic goals.

Efficiency in work and sports is but one criterion of health among others. It is a maximin concept in the sense of translating health as a maximal efficiency and effectiveness with minimal

---

[1] Viktor von Weizsaecker, Diesseits und jenseits der Medizin (Stuttgart, 1951), p. 196.

fatigue and weariness — a condition which, to a great extent, is contingent on proper training, reasonable diet and a wholesome life-style. The last decades have provided increasing evidence that one's overall well-being depends greatly on the quality of the environment and on social stimulation. Where general efficiency is of a particularly high level, social recognition plays a commanding rôle.[2]

Different from productive efficiency and athletic stamina is the capacity to confront difficult life situations without loss of stability and without significant impairment of bodily and mental health. This definition of health points to a man's vitality in the unswerving pursuit of worthy cultural acquirements and spiritual attainments.

Health cannot be defined from a mere study of the body; we must consider the whole person in his human vocation and final destiny. A comprehensive understanding of human health includes the greatest possible harmony of all of man's forces and energies, the greatest possible spiritualization of man's bodily aspect and the finest embodiment of the spiritual. True health is revealed in the self-actualization of the person who has attained that freedom which marshals all available energies for the fulfilment of his total human vocation.

Purely physiological health, viewed as exuberant vitality and freedom from pain, is too narrow and even too dangerous a concept; it would suitably describe the health of animals. This limited definition of health may actually stunt human well-being in its full sense since it reveals and promotes a lamentable imbalance and under-development of man as an embodied spirit. A bubbling bodily vitality which oppresses the spirit comes closer to sickness than does a relatively feeble body, compliant to the spirit and truly subservient to that freedom which is the principal condition and precious fruit of a growing love of God and of one's neighbour. Such a ranking of values does not suggest contempt for human vitality or disdain of bodily strength

---

[2] Hans Schäfer, 'Probleme der Leistungsfährgkeit des Menschen,' *Arzt und Christ*, 12 (1966), 207-215.

and robustness; it does not preclude joyousness flowing from bodily well-being. What is disavowed is the making absolute of sheer physical vitality, since this is not a holistically human vitality but one inferior to it. The robust, well-trained and energetic body, toughened and supple, which is an expression and instrument of the spirit and a manifestation of freedom, has a high value.

The ups and downs of physical strength may sometimes contribute notably more to the total growth of the person than an unrestrained vitality. Obviously, mere bodily health is far less significant than psychological and spiritual health; we must be mindful, however, of the dependence of psychological conditions on the integrity and soundness of bodily organs.

If death looms as the greatest of all evils, the prolongation of life, even at the cost of a diminished or somewhat suppressed freedom, seems to be imperative. Our conception of life and death suggests that we aim for that kind of health that would allow the best possible fulfilment of man's total vocation regardless of time. 'Human life is misunderstood if there is interest only in the number of years and if medical care includes only the condition of the body.' [3]

For each person and his doctor, health is not an abstraction but a desirable reality. Each individual person has to maintain *his* health with its inherited potential and limitations. The most decisive factor is the person's degree of charity and the depth with which he envisages health and accepts it as a means of attaining his destiny. The disciple of Christ is willing to risk his health in the service of others whenever this is reasonable.

2. *Health and the pursuit of holiness*

The ancient Romans prayed for 'a sound mind in a sound body,' but the healthy mind is not necessarily a function of bodily strength. How many healthy souls are in sick and feeble

---

[3] J.H. Van den Berg, *The Psychology of the Sickbed* (Penn.: Duquesne University Press, 1966), p. 57.

bodies and how many sick souls in healthy bodies! Saint
Hildegard and Tauler assert that, 'A healthy body is not usually
the dwelling place of God or, as Saint Paul tells us, power comes
to its full strength in weakness (II Cor 12:9).' 'This,' it is added,
'does not usually result from external ascetical practices but
from the overwhelming outpouring of the Godhead, which
floods a person so powerfully that the poor body cannot endure
it.' [4] A total commitment to God and neighbour in the following
of Christ, a whole-hearted search for truth with the prospect
of living it can be staggering at times, ruffling one's usual
equanimity. But it is equally true that, in the end, a profound and
healthy effect derives from it.[5]

The experience of the mystics attests to the scriptural truth
that no one can see God and live (Ex 33:20). Saint John of
the Cross holds that a deep mystical experience of God's holiness,
if it were suddenly to overwhelm a non-purified person, would
have something deadly about it. Even the purification by which
God gradually prepares man for his saving presence is very
painful, although it simultaneously grants a new experience of
the magnetizing and blissful mystery of his love and the
beatitude of serving him in his children.

A growing existential knowledge of God unsettles one's
shallow security and, like an earthquake, uncovers the hitherto
hidden lives of men. To the selfish ego, this means dread and
anguish, but it eventually leads to better health. Something
analogous is happening in the Church today with the loss of
that superficial security founded on laws and formulations which
once spelled salvation. There is a great deal of pain until the
new situation is understood and accepted. Its meaning must
be probed with absolute sincerity in the face of life's problems
and it will be found through trust in God.

Salvation and holiness have much to do with the wholeness
and health of the human person, but for sinning man the path

---

[4] Cited by J. Bernhart, 'Heiligkeit und Krankheit,' *Geist und Leben*,
23 (1950), 177.
[5] *Ibid.*, p. 185.

leads through a painful purification. Whoever is unwilling to expose his shallow earthly security and health to pain and risk — obviously, within the bounds of prudence — in view of greater union with God and a more generous commitment to fraternal love, will never become holy nor reach a fully human, redeemed health. I wish however, to make this point clear: whoever squanders his health by exposing it foolishly, be it even through false asceticism or a self-centred and unnatural form of recollection and prayer, risks both his sanctity and his sanity. The road to holiness is paved with genuinely prudent concern for health in view of authentic love and growth in this love, and a humble readiness to accept the human predicament of illness.

3. *The sense and nonsense of illness*

The definition of illness follows that of health. Sickness as a diminution of efficiency and a dysfunction of organs is a deviation from the anatomic-physiological or psychological norm. The personal experience of it reveals the frailty of human existence. Man has illnesses but, to some extent, we can say that he creates his ailments, and above all gives them meaning. In various forms and degrees, illness has its personal structure. Acquaintance with the biography of a person, his life experiences and the way he confronts diverse human situations can often help us to understand his malady.[6]

As a being committed to death, man must indeed tread his way to his eternal goal through death's doors and varying degrees of sickness. 'Illness belongs to human existence.'[7] It reveals our human frailty and can thus be a blessed experience by refocusing our pilgrim's vision on the imperishable life, and bidding us reflect more deeply on the profound truths of our existence. In times of illness, we are urged 'to assess again the perils that beset us and to recognize again our human destiny

---

[6] Cf.: K. Gastgeber, 'Vom Sinn der Krankheit,' *Arzt und Christ*, 15 (1969), 90.

[7] V. von Weizsaecker, *Diesseits, op. cit.*, p. 199.

and vocation.' [8] But before illness befalls a person, he should prepare himself to face it and to decipher its meaning in the context of life and salvation.

It would be naïve to think that by itself illness is a means of salvation. On the whole, the medical profession has good reasons for considering it an evil to be combated and eventually eliminated. Often it points to sin, though not necessarily to personal or individual sin; in a great many illnesses we bear the burden of the guilt and failures of our ancestors. Our genetic heritage is a bearer of frailty and of burdensome traits and qualities; there can be harmful prenatal disturbances and sicknesses, childhood accidents, polluted air and water, the stress of life, the daily sensory overload from our technotronic world (for example, the blaring radio or television, the urban traffic din, the monotonous grind of automated equipment), the negligence or malice of our fellowmen, the institutionalized temptations — altogether these tax man's physical and psychical endurance beyond his level of tolerance.

Disease is often enough the consequence and manifestation of personal sin, be it in the context of violent outbursts, intemperance, drug abuse or impurity, all of which can be quick to avenge themselves. Each sin is in some way an attack on 'health.' Man cannot attain wholeness and peace if he refuses to act on his best insights and on his inborn longing for light and dedication to truth and justice. The person who severs himself from God, the source of truth, goodness and life, is dissociated from the ground of his being and alienated from the saving relationship with God's creation.

The burden of sin weighs heavily upon the centre of man's life touching as it does that innermost point where all his faculties either experience complete harmony or suffer from inner disruption. The violation of a person's conscience sunders his spiritual unity. We speak here of sin in its existential sense and of the consequence of sin which encodes and records misleading

---

[8] *Ibid.*

'information' in the cerebral cortex, in the depths of the psyche, in man's total being and in a more and more disturbed world. All this is particularly true if a person neglects the speedy healing of the spirit through sorrow and reparation with respect to the disturbed order.

Among representatives of the anthropological school of medicine, Weizsaecker incessantly reminds us of the inadequacy of a purely biochemical explanation of illness: 'Disease has formed itself upon us as a critic of human life and human relationships. We can no longer avoid confronting it as a touchstone of human conduct and behaviour.'[9] 'As far as we have been able to establish up to now, the outbreak and development of certain infectious diseases has much to do with the moral situation of a man but practically nothing to do with his cultural activities. Similarly, in a host of other diseases, such as circulatory troubles and metabolic dysfunctions, it is unmistakably evident how closely the biological chain of their development is bound up with erotic or moral crises, which can also be chronic.'[10]

It has often been observed how tuberculosis, from inception to crisis, reflects serious failures or disappointments in love, a family tragedy or other fateful experience, the direst of all being one's own moral failure or that of persons close to oneself. In some cases, sickness manifests a tendency to punish oneself.[11] An interesting phenomenon related to this is the 'executive illness' (Manager *Krankheit*). People entrapped in the process of management, unable to vent their emotions and to enjoy life in itself, show a predisposition to certain diseases.[12] In a number of cases, people say intuitively, 'He has escaped into illness.'[13] But even in such cases, we are far from justified in judging the sick person; it may well be that the situational demands exceeded

---

[9] *Ibid.*, p. 104.

[10] *Ibid.*, p. 107.

[11] P. Tournier, *Krankheit und Lebensprobleme* (Basel, 1965), pp. 80 ff.

[12] *Ibid.*, pp. 117 ff.

[13] *Ibid.*, p. 102. Also: E. Stern, *Arzt und Patient in der Gegenwart* (München-Basel, 1958), pp. 31 ff.

L

his moral and psychic energies. An increasing number of illness biographies give special attention to the stress of living with difficult people in a congested milieu.

While I accept for many cases a more or less tangible relationship between sickness and sin in one dimension or another, I would strongly object to any over-generalization. 'Illness cannot automatically be brought into relation with personal guilt, since human nature is extremely vulnerable to the environment. There are diseases which man causes (the illness of the anthropological school of medicine) and there are others to which man is subjected (the illness of the classical schools of medicine).' [14]

4. Illness and temptation

For the physician and the nurse, for friends and the hospital chaplain, it is especially important to be alert to the dangers and temptations besetting a patient in conjunction with his illness. Sickness itself and the particular situation of estrangement in the hospital environment often have profound psychological repercussions and may even cause personality changes and identity crises.[15] In most cases, an awareness on the part of all persons involved can reduce the risks and even transform them into positive opportunities for growth. Most commonly there is not so much a problem of actual change in the total personality structure as a gradual shift that brings specific weaknesses boldly into prominence. Nevertheless, some special instances as in diseases of the lungs and stomach have been observed to induce deep changes of attitudes and behaviour affecting the whole of personality and character.[16]

---

[14] R. Kautzky, 'Die Bedentung der Person des Menschen in der modernen medizinischen Wissenschaft,' *Arzt und Christ,* 10 (1964), 172.

[15] Cf.: A. Guirdham, *Krankheit als Schicksal* (Freiburg/Br., 1960), p. 112. H. Fleckenstein, *Persönlichkeit und Organminderwertigkeiten* (Freiburg/Br., 1938). E. Erikson, *Insight and Responsibility* (N.Y.: W.W. Norton, 1964), p. 97.

[16] Cf.: P. Bolech, 'Das Bild des kranken Menschen,' *Arzt und Christ,* 15 (1969), 100.

Strong *insecurity and anguish* is likely to assail the patient suffering from a chronic disease.[17] While fear arises in confrontation with an actual danger or pain, it is rational and focalized; anxiety, on the other hand, is characterized by a general and pervasive state of apprehensiveness and sadness. Anguish cannot muster energies to overcome its disquietude; just the opposite, it paralyzes constructive energies so that all psychic reactions are negatively impressed. The degree and form of the anxious response vary not only with the temperament and character of the sufferer but also with his social environment.[18]

Anguish is generally caused or occasioned by inactivity and alienation from normal life, inferiority complexes, diminished energy and freedom. Hospitalization can be traumatic if the patient unwillingly experiences its quiet strangeness and the impersonal trappings of the whole situation: an all too bureaucratic reception, proximity to restless, apprehensive and depressed patients, to which are added feelings of self-pity flowing from the inappropriate attitude of visitors who do not know how to meet and comfort the sick person.

Inferiority complexes thrive on the devaluation intimated by the impersonal and depersonalizing attitudes of various specialists and technicians, the long waiting for medical examinations or procedures, and the policy of doctors and nurses in deceiving the patient about his true situation. The lessened efficiency, the waning beauty and unattractive attire, exposure to a misguided compassion, fear of contaminating or burdening others, the uncertainty of the future — all contribute to cause or deepen feelings of personal inadequacy. The gradual loss of physical strength needed for freedom of action, the humbling dependence on others, restricted social contacts, the inability to fulfil his family *rôle* — all have a cumulative effect in bringing the patient to the point of losing his *freedom to hope*. Total depression ensues which can even give rise to thoughts of suicide.

---

[17] Cf.: P. Valdigivé, 'La psychologie du malade,' *Cahiers Albert le Grand*, 29 (1954), 13-25.

[18] P. Tournier, *Krankheit, op. cit.*, pp. 74 ff.

Hypersensitivity and irritability can be other by-products of the patient's debilitating situation. The central nervous system may be markedly weakened by the adverse and toxic effects of medication, while pain, heightened excitability, sleeplessness, heart disturbances and indigestion may add still further to his discomfort. If the patient's irritability antagonizes those about him to the point where they strongly express their displeasure, he faces growing difficulty in achieving peace and balance.

At times, the lability of the patient's affective life is totally unexpected and may even seem unwarranted. It is not unusual for adult patients occasionally to regress to a certain infantilism or to emotional reactions properly adolescent. Lack of self-control, obstinacy, egocentrism, morbid concern for bodily health and in some cases pure hypochondria, thanklessness and resentment towards the nurse and doctor may develop in patients who exhibit great self-restraint and emotional control when in better health.

Some patients experience anguish over increasing erotic desires and sexual tensions; this can happen particularly in cases of pulmonary affections.[19] It may be accounted for by the convergence of all attention on the body, the inactivity which gives free rein to the fantasy world, suggestive reading, and possibly arousal as a secondary effect of medication. The diminution of the psychosomatic energies, the lessened resistance, the enforced confinement can lead to a dangerous *abulia* (want of will) which can defeat convalescence.[20]

In view of all these complicating factors, it is most important to find the golden mean between a moralistic 'judgmental' attitude and a fatalistic acceptance of the situation as unavoidable. Doctor and patient should learn to discriminate between aspects and dimensions which must be accepted and those calling for change. It is a question of operating judiciously within the given limitations of freedom and responsibility.

---

[19] Fr. Székély, TBC, *Seelische Probleme und ihre Uberwindung* (Wien, 1957).
[20] Cf.: P. Tournier, *Krankheit, op. cit.*, pp. 89 ff.

The sacrament of the anointing of the sick implores God's grace for this particularly trying moment of life. It is a time when the person concerned needs all the comforting power of the Good News, supportive understanding, supportive effective motivation and discernment of the gravity of his situation. Doctor and nurse are often the key persons to communicate to the patient the needed insights and motives.

While recognizing that a time of illness can be a time of temptation, our primary focus should be on the spiritual opportunities inherent in it. The very *kairos* of temptation in times of illness can prove to be a privileged moment in the history of the patient's personal liberty. He can experience his creaturely frailty to the point of feeling a greater need for humility, for total trust in God's mercy and healing kindness. He can also become more understanding of his fellowmen. The school of suffering in a setting of enforced inactivity is an urgent appeal to attain greater depth, to set a new and clearer direction for one's whole life.

5. Sinful failure to accept the meaning of illness

Obviously, the causes of illness are many and varied, and its meaning can be manifold, but the decisive factor lies in the sick person's sincere quest for the personal message in his illness and for the real possibilities offered and suggested by it for the reorientation of his life. The greatest failure would be the patient's refusal to ask himself what message is concealed in his sickness or defiantly to close his mind to it and allow himself to become passive or resentful.

Later, in our discussion of neurosis and its treatment, I shall give special attention to those psychosomatic ailments which, by their whole structure, appeal urgently for more than symptomatic relief of bodily ills. With the indispensable assistance of a competent doctor, the patient's effort to regain true health will lead to a lessening or eradication of the complex defensive system which camouflages the root of the illness.

Whatever may be the cause of ill-health (perhaps personal guilt), illness always offers a favourable opportunity to those who believe in redemption. If the sick person earnestly looks for the meaning of health and sickness in his life, he already begins to transcend himself. It is because of the human predicament that the patient relies on the assistance of others in this all-important quest. If he can accept this help, he opens himself to a new experience of human solidarity. When the incidence of illness reveals human frailty and unmasks partial immaturity, then one of its chief messages is this very knowledge of self which exhorts to a deeper conversion. I would like to insist on the fact that it is not so much the illness itself that causes the notorious self-centredness of the sick, but rather a case of sickness exposing an already existent egocentrism and thus offering a new chance for conversion.[21]

If illness spells the painful experience of restricted freedom and incapacitation, it can nevertheless insert itself positively into the history of personal liberation. The sick person who capitalizes on the opportunity gains beneficial self-knowledge and a new freedom by accepting his human dependence on God's grace and the help of others. Many diseases have nothing or little to do with the patient's personal guilt, yet they can lead to a deep personal experience of solidarity with sinful mankind. The man purified by pain and suffering learns to be compassionate towards a troubled humanity. Sin may begin precisely where the sick person refuses this unfolding message and rejects the opportunity for authentic growth in freedom by his hankering and attitude of 'if only. . . .'

Illness *per se* has to be seen primarily as a disorder, a chaotic interference with creation; but in that freedom which arises from faith in redemption, the patient and his doctor can fight this chaos and transform the seemingly meaningless into a creative and redeeming event. Illness then becomes an appeal to silence the self-centred ego and to enter more fully into the realm of the freedom of God's children who, *in faith,* place their total trust in him precisely at the moment when their difficulties

---

[21] Fr. Pastorelli, *Servitude et grandeur de la maladie* (Paris, 1967), pp. 145-150.

offer no possibility of self-trust. The true Christian will finally try to see adversity in the light of the paschal mystery.[22] Suffering thus accepted gives a new dimension to life and announces the approach of life everlasting.

6. Redemption and healing

Illness seen in the light of the paschal mystery prevents both the patient and the doctor from focusing one-sidedly on suffering. The mystery of redemption draws the doctor to the one Redeemer and Healer, for his curative efforts are directed towards the restoration and development of his patient's freedom, and towards the finding of meaning in life and death through increasing altruistic love and service. All of the doctor's decisions and attitudes towards the patient are then governed by this view of redemptive liberation integrated with wisdom and a holistic vision. The sick person, on his part, accepts the healing of his bodily and psychic ailments as a symbol and promise of final redemption and liberation.[23]

The whole gospel confirms the thesis that illness is not to be seen solely in a mystique of suffering. It presents Christ primarily as Healer and Liberator; for he considered curing the sick essential to his mission (Cf.: Lk 4: 16-22; Mt 11: 2-6). The repeated healing of sick persons on the sabbath symbolizes the urgency of restoring them to health; it indicates that man's sabbath, that is, his repose and peace in God, has a healing quality. Already the prophets had described the Messianic age as one of peace and of healing of the sick (Cf.: Is 61: 1-3; Mich 4: 1-4; Jer 33: 6). Christ's healing power, however, did not presage absolute earthly happiness and health; he preferred directing attention towards the final fulfilment of redemption.

---

[22] S. Spinsanti, 'Il cristiano e la malattia alla luce della morale Pasquale,' *Anime e corpi*, 32 (1970), 345-365.

[23] Cf.: E. Mark Stern and Bert G. Marino, *Psychotheology* (N.Y.: Newman Press, 1970). Cf. also: Elizabeth O'Connor, *Our Many Selves* (New York: Harper and Row, 1971).

The healing of the sick has to be viewed in the light of Jesus' choice of the way of suffering and death in order to reveal the resurrection and final redemption. The mission of the Divine Physician and his personal acceptance of suffering and death must be seen in their thorough interrelatedness. The sick person approaches redemption if he seeks to heal what can be healed and accepts in love what cannot.

If, by faith, sickness is inserted into the sacrificial love of Christ, then despite and even through its frustrating experiences, it can be a way towards redemption and freedom. The help of others assumes importance here. The circumstances of illness call upon the Christian to act as a Christian specifically in those situations where overcoming egotism would be impossible without a strong faith. The sick person will keep himself from narrowness of vision and egocentric concern over his own predicament if he models his whole life on Christ, who manifestly lived the fidelity of the covenant in his passion, the consummate sign of solidarity. By increasingly cooperating with the doctor, the patient can seek healing for what can be healed, but at the same time, his true freedom receives its greatest increase through his accepting in faith the limits of his healing.[24]

Christ finally liberated all the energies of love through the acceptance of death in solidarity and compassion. For a believer, the part of illness which has to be accepted can thus inspire final trust in God. However, for healing and acceptance of what cannot be healed to become sacramental signs of liberation, there must be dialogue between God who alone can save and man who is longing for redemption. Both by prayer and by recourse to medical resources man recognizes the healing and redeeming action of Christ in the whole history of salvation. Whoever can enter into this perspective when beset by illness becomes a witness to faith in loving gratitude and in renewed compassion towards others.

---

[24] Cf.: G. Crespy, *La guérison par la foi* (Neuchâtel, 1952).

B. *Psychopathology and psychotherapy*

In the field of psychopathology, everything points to Pilate's question: 'what is truth?' Applied to medicine, it becomes: what is truly human health? what is the goal of therapy?[25] The humanistic branch of psychotherapy and particularly logotherapy turn all their attention to this fundamental question and thereby contribute substantially to the whole of medicine. Each patient is seen in his irreplaceable uniqueness and in his singular situation. It thus becomes easier for modern medicine to differentiate the various phenomena of illness.

1. *Psychopathology: neurosis-psychosis*

Neurosis (or psychoneurosis) entails suffering on the psychic level and therefore belongs to the generic classification of psychopathology. The terminology and distinctions tend to be fluid, and this all the more so since modern medicine is now reluctant to distinguish sharply between illnesses deemed inherited and incurable and those caused by the environment and therefore amenable to treatment. Neurosis is generally considered an acquired illness but, to a great extent, it builds on genetic predispositions.

The main distinction between psychosis and other psychopathologies lies in the psychotic's inability to gain distance from his sickness; he cannot discern mental impairment from the domain of freedom and responsibility. In other cases of psychological dysfunction, a certain degree of freedom remains and, above all, the sick person retains some, albeit limited, capacity to discriminate between the games of his psychopathology and his personal decisions. He can gain distance from his anomaly and the therapist will focus attention particularly on this point. However, the classical clear-cut distinction between psychosis and other psychopathologies is becoming blurred as progress in

---

[25] Viktor E. Frankl, *Arztliche Seelsorge* (7th ed.), (Wien: Franz Deutsche, 1966), p. 1. English version: *The Doctor and the Soul* (London: Souvenir Press, 1969).

psychiatry increases the possibility of helping psychotic patients reach the point where they can discriminate and gain distance.

More important is the distinction between endogenous, psychogenic and nöogenic disturbances.[26] There is a great difference between an endogenous depression and a psychogenic depression, between a depressive psychosis and depressive neurosis. Depending on the different etiology and various phenomena, the treatment will differ considerably although today there are transitions between psychiatry and psychotherapy and combinations of the two which were not so apparent twenty years ago.

A neurosis sums up the patient's life history and points primarily to early childhood experiences. It arises from an unsuccessful attempt to meet the difficulties of life or from a lack of courage to do so. To a considerable extent, neurosis is a product of the environment, for psychic health-sickness reflects achievements or failures bound to a social context; they never occur in a vacuum. Man is a responsorial, dialogical being whose dialectical relationship depends on all persons with whom he interacts. The burden of responsibility for the neurotic condition may rest with others as much as with the victim of neurosis. A person who constantly fails to adjust to the reality of his life and environment, or one who is so overburdened by his life situation that he is unable to turn to good account a failure, a personal trial, a tragedy or a material loss grows sick in his whole existential rapport with himself and the world about him.

'A neurosis affects a person who is in a state of unresolved conflict and yet is unconsciously pressured towards a healing change. It appears that, under the given circumstances, it is better to be affected by a neurosis than to be beaten and flung about as the plaything of uncontrolled forces in subhuman inarticulateness. Of course, a neurotic resolves an existential

---

[26] *Endogenous, arising from within the body; psychogenic,* of mental origin, as opposed to *somatogenic,* of organic etiology; *nöogenic,* existential in origin, for example, related to values, meaningfulness.

problem on a level lower than the one on which it is situated.' [27]
'One of the most important characteristics of neurosis is that it
develops and grows out of the unconscious. There is no neurosis
which springs up and develops in the full light of conscious
awareness.' [28] Like most illnesses of psychogenic origin, it arises
from the repression of unresolved experiences of stress which
have been at least partially rejected and shelved in the subconscious. In final analysis, it is an illness of the embodied
spirit's failure to find its own significance and integration, while
in the very depths of the unconscious the person is still searching
for meaning.

Psychology warns that a moralistic or 'judgmental' attitude
towards neurotics can be a grave mistake; it can even constitute
a most harmful injustice to them. Among morally obtuse persons
with a totally undeveloped sensitivity, neurosis does not readily
occur; for the robust 'health' of these people eliminates the need
for repression.

Neurosis is never simply or generally reducible to sin or to
personal guilt. However, it is somewhat analogous to the outcry
of conscience whose continued violation brings about illness, a
dreadful disintegration in the innermost depths of the person.
But while the clamour of conscience is a conscious longing for
healing, neurosis remains on the subconscious plane although
manifesting itself in a series of discernible symptoms. It can
result from a failure to search consciously for the healing of
conscience's wound: in this way the disturbance and the longing
for a radical cure are repressed into the subconscious level of
psychic life ('refoulement').

According to the logotherapeutic school of Viktor Frankl,
about twenty per cent of all psychoneuroses today develop in an
'existential vacuum,' that is, the existential predicament of the
person who finds no meaning or significance in his life. It seems
that there is a mounting incidence of 'nöogenic' neuroses in a

---

[27] V. von Weizsaecker, *Diesseits, op. cit.*, p. 64.
[28] E. Speer, *Vom Wesen der Neurose* (Stuttgart, 1949), p. 23.

materialistic welfare society. The 'existential vacuum' is often nothing less than the collective neurosis of the whole entourage, of a social environment devoid of sense and ideals. The 'hippie' condemns this meaningless emptiness and breaks out of his family and immediate cultural milieu to search for new albeit strange communications. Typical neurosis, on the other hand, plays a concealed hand on the unconscious level. Where the hippies are groping in their thrust towards selfhood, the neurotic remains stationary, a psychological cripple chained by unconscious defences.

In seeking to explain the nature of neurosis, Jung constantly refers to man's deep religious disposition and to his longing for a life fulfilled in love, the neglect of which avenges itself somehow in the depths of the human personality. Neurotic illness befalls man as a consequence of an unfulfilled life only because in his innermost being he has not renounced significance, love and integration. That is why it is asserted that a totally blunted or insensitive nature would not be affected by neurosis but that its 'health' would be no more than animal vitality. Under certain circumstances, it can be shown that 'health conceals a deep misery (*Unheilstiefe*) of the soul and hence is not really healthy at its roots.' [29]

It is commonly agreed that neuroses and all psychogenic illnesses have potential value despite all the hazards involved. At a more profound level they can be compared to a fever which simultaneously reveals illness and organizes the bodily forces to overcome it. The neurotic person harbours, deep in the unconscious self, a sense of being called to fulfilment. The suffering caused by neurosis recounts the basic effort of the soul to uncover its misery and resume a new and more significant existence. When rightly understood, these psychogenic illnesses can disclose a humbling truth and summon the sufferer to the truth of life.

---

[29] V. von Gebsattel, *Christentum und Humanismus* (Stuttgart, 1947), p. 53.

2. *Psychosomatic illness*

To cling to a unilateral and even materialistic biochemical concept of medicine today would be anachronistic in view of our recognition of the psychosomatic nature of so many illnesses. There are ailments to be healed by pharmacological means and many others that need a more holistic approach. The modern physician is therefore obliged to acquire competence in diagnosing differentially the somatogenic and the psychogenic ailment. This implies sufficient psychological knowledge for a physician to recognize when he should refer his patient to a competent psychotherapist. No less should the psychotherapist know the limits of his own discipline and methods.

Teamwork between the general practitioner and the psychotherapist is a promising development in medicine today. Very often the specialist in internal medicine will be more competent to discern endogenic pseudo-neuroses and treat them with the classical means of medicine. Teamwork will be facilitated if both the general practitioner and the psychotherapist have the basic knowledge of man's psychosomatic reality. In many cases, an experienced practitioner with a sound knowledge of psychology can, in a relaxed conversation, unravel psychic knots. Cooperation however does not mean intrusion. An inexperienced and insufficiently knowledgeable practitioner who trespasses into the field of psychoanalysis can cause great harm. The same situation exists in other medical specialities when a doctor blinds himself to the limits of his competence. In the psychoanalytic realm, however, the risk is even greater because the psychic and mental health of the person is in jeopardy.

Continuing education through participation in courses and extensive professional reading can enable physicians to assemble their own anamnetic biography. This would indeed be helpful since there is little hope that a great number of physicians will find time and energy to undergo psychoanalysis, although this could result in great gains in professional efficiency and in personal self-knowledge. Jores recommends group therapy for doctors, surmising that the common disclosure of their failures and limitations in medical practice would help all the participants, particularly in physician-patient relationships.[30] Beyond such knowledge, his own personal balance, his absolute respect for his patients, and his capacity for good relations with them will bear importantly on the efficacy of a doctor's daily ministrations. By his very vocation, each physician has to strive for an organismic knowledge of man in order to serve the total health of his patients, but the physician should always heed the wisdom of the words of Paracelsus: 'The best medicine is loving respect.'

3. Psychoanalysis and logotherapy

Teilhard de Chardin sees the finality of hominization in the development of the highest possible form of conscious awareness. In no way, however, does he think of a vague, introspective consciousness centred in the egotistic self. To him Christ is the point Omega of consciousness through his supremely conscious awareness of the Father and of his own mission, namely, that of being sent to all his brothers and sisters, to all men of all nations. The whole groping of creation springs from its dynamism towards this kind of consciousness.

(a) Psychoanalysis

The constructs of Sigmund Freud can, in this respect, be considered as very important although of limited breadth and depth. He detected the groping of the subconscious psychic life but not its point Omega. It is only through a breakthrough of the subconscious into the realm of consciousness that healing is possible for those illnesses caused by repression. Freud limits his vision to the subconscious storage of repressions without fully integrating the unconscious into the total groping for consciousness in love.

Whatever may be said against the *Weltanschauung* which serves as the background of many of Freud's interpretations, it cannot be denied that through the psychological study of the

[30] Arthur Jores, *Vom kranken Menschen* (Stuttgart, 1960).

subconscious, our knowledge of man and our means of healing are greatly extended. The goal of Freud's psychoanalysis is to enlarge the space of the ego by liberating those realities or experiences which are imprisoned in the 'id'. He wants to eliminate what is restricting the ego as ego by bringing as much as possible of the unconscious sphere into the conscious. Through analysis, man becomes aware of the libidinal character of all his unconscious strivings, and, indeed, of all his life as swayed by unconscious repressions. Adler's school of 'individual psychology' tends to override Freud's undue restriction on the ego by positing a 'will-to-power.' This Adlerian construct enables the ego to assume responsibility and to channel its dynamism towards power by operating in and through the unconscious. These two viewpoints which have so often opposed one another could greatly profit by considering their basic complementarity.

(b) *Logotherapy*

The tendencies towards materialistic abuse of psychoanalytic methods are counteracted today by impressive efforts to re-humanize psychotherapy. Such valiant contributions have come from no less than Carl Jung and Viktor von Gebsattel. I mention them specifically because of my indebtedness to them although I am cognizant of the fact that many others would likewise deserve attention. In this section, I shall be guided particularly by Viktor Frankl's logotherapy which promises to gain a great following.[31]

As Frankl points out time and again, he does not intend to replace psychoanalysis by logotherapy. His concern centres on the need for sharper diagnostic distinctions in order to rule out the somatogenic pseudo-neuroses which call for biochemical treatment and to focus on the endogenous psychopathologies requiring the expertise of psychiatry and clinical psychology. Frankl gives particular attention to the nöogenic neurosis which he predicts will be the 'neurosis of the future.' 'The great

---

[31] See extensive bibliography in Frankl, *Ärztliche Seelsorge, op. cit.,* pp. 257-264.

sickness of our age is aimlessness, boredom, lack of meaning and purpose.'[32] An example is the 'Sunday neurosis': the neurotic condition of people who fear nothing more than having to reflect on Sundays, and so escape into ever new diversions.

When psychoanalysis does not help the patient to find meaning and purpose in life, it deals with symptoms only without penetrating the depths of the nöogenic neurosis. For Frankl and his school, the cardinal point of treatment rests with existential analysis, the twofold purpose of which is to free man in his search for life's meaning and to bolster or enlarge his capacity to assume his unique responsibility.

Like the whole stream of psychoanalysis the logotherapeutic school recognizes the importance of transference, but Frankl gives it full personalistic direction by considering it a vehicle of existential encounter in which the patient finds the realization of his dialogical, responsorial existence. Freud sees love only as a by-product or epiphenomenon of human life; Frankl, on the contrary, asserts that the ego becomes thoroughly 'I' uniquely through its encounter with the 'Thou' as 'Thou'. Only the 'I' that intends to open itself to the world and to its fellowmen in self-transcendence can integrate the 'id' into its conscious life.

While psychoanalysis often deems it sufficient to elevate the psychic sphere to consciousness, logotherapy guides to a fuller consciousness by directing attention to the spiritual domain, to personal responsibility, to the significance and value of the human vocation. It grounds human existence in the capacity to listen to the needs of one's fellowmen and to respond to them.[35] The doors to mental health swing outwards. 'True neuroses are best defined as stubborn self-centredness. No therapist can cure a phobia, obsession or prejudice by subtraction. He can assist the patient to achieve a value system and outlook that can blanket or absorb the troublesome factor.' [34]

---

[32] *Ibid.*, p. 5.
[33] *Ibid., op. cit.*, p. 39.
[34] Gordon W. Allport, *Personality and Social Encounter* (Boston: Beacon Press, 1960), p. 173.

Logotherapy does not indulge in abstract preaching about meaning; it demands a respectful meeting of the patient in his need. For that purpose, logotherapy has elaborated effective techniques in order to liberate man from unhealthy imprisonment in his self-made defensive system. One such technique is the 'paradoxical intention.' [35] The effectiveness of the device is supported by that kind of humour which allows the patient to view himself objectively and not take himself too seriously while simultaneously experiencing the trust and respect of the therapist.

The sense of humour allows the patient to gain distance from his anguish, obsession or phobia, and to make it an object of laughter — something alien to him — by a jocularity which finds expression in the paradoxical intention. For instance, if a patient is immobilized by a phobic conviction that he will collapse on the street, he is taught to humour himself by saying at each step, 'Now I want to collapse!' Very often, after a few sessions only, the patient will smilingly admit that he is no longer able to identify with the fear of collapsing. The same method can also be applied for insomnia and similar problems. The paradoxical intention is meant to transcend the neurotic fixation. It can therefore be of instrumental value in the healing process where the person learns to transcend his egocentrism in the search for meaning and purpose. So the technique operates exclusively within logotherapy.

It must be emphasized, however, that an application of the technique presupposes an accurate diagnosis. In the case of an endogenous depressive neurosis or other somatogenic psychopathologies, for example, where the patient is plagued by suicidal compulsions, the application of the 'paradoxical intention' technique would be a grave mistake.[36] Quite different is the effect of this logotherapeutic method in treating cases of psychogenic, nöogenic obsession or phobia, where the kernel of the phenomenon lies in the expectation of the difficulty (*Erwartungsangst*).

---

[35] V. Frankl, *Arztliche Seelsorge, op. cit.*, p. 194.
[36] *Ibid.*, pp. 242 ff.

M

(c) *The dangers of psychoanalysis*

The humanistic branch of psychotherapy points out the dangers and temptations inherent in certain schools of psychoanalysis.

(1) Psychoanalysis often asserts its independence from all value systems while in reality the whole treatment implies a definite *Weltanschauung*. It thus operates under a most insidious repression, namely, a denial in consciousness of its own outlook and direction. The repressed *Weltanschauung,* the carefully veiled and smothered quest for the meaning of health, unhealthily breaks through like any other kind of repression and plays its concealed game. Humanistic psychotherapy, on the other hand, and particularly Frankl's logotherapeutic school, works out a concept of human existence and of human health in absolute consciousness and frankness. It does not allow itself to repress or to suppress the question although it is fully aware that solutions and answers are not always readily available. Frankl strongly emphasizes that the search for meaning and purpose remains always the responsibility of this unique person. The logotherapist will therefore scrupulously avoid any kind of concession just as he will refrain from imposing his own religious faith or conviction. He meets his patient as a man seeking freedom through the pursuit of truth and meaning.

(2) A second danger of psychoanalysis comes from transference, a phenomenon which often turns into an unjust and harmful manipulation of the patient. The danger is even greater because of the repressed nature of the patient's quest for the meaning of life which recurs constantly as a target for the manipulative handling of the transference. Thus the therapeutic session, including the dependent transference relationship, will fail to attain the level of common search for meaning and true love. The therapist will then easily impose his own domination (though repressed) through manipulative concessions on the lower level of the libidinal *Weltanschauung* or even on that of power. Besides the failure to liberate the patient for his own freedom, there may have been an intrusion into the personality to the point of a change in identity.

(3) A third danger lurking in some psychoanalytic models is that, consciously or not, they revolve around an individualistic concept of man. This pivotal weakness is part and parcel of the collective neuroses of self-centredness, and gives rise to an egotistic brand of personalism. It is readily acknowledged today that many neuroses have their roots in a navel-gazing type of introspection, in total attention to one's ego. For instance, in many neuroses, the principal cause is the unhealthy attention given to one's body in narcissistic and pleasure-seeking attitudes. If, through transference and beyond it, the meaning of life is found in an encounter of the Thou-We-I, only then can the real existential realm of the 'I' be enlarged and the person attain freedom. He will then find fulfilment in a significant purpose.

Psychoanalysis of the Freudian stamp overemphasizes the *libido,* the search for pleasure and happiness. Max Scheler, whom Frankl often quotes, demonstrated that the empty seeking of pleasure and happiness is condemned to existential frustration. Only in reaching out for meaning through dedication to others and in acceptance of a scale of values can man find his true happiness and fulfilment. The *libido* concept of Freud militates against this holistic vision. In fact, the therapeutic approach of many psychoanalysts hinges so much on the *libido* that personal growth is thoroughly blocked, and treatment can go on for years and years.

(4) A further danger is detected when we realize that neuroses and psychogenic illnesses are frequently characterized by *escapism,* a certain flight from responsibility in the face of the difficulties and tensions of life. If psychoanalysis is totally embedded in the *libido* concept, there is a grave danger that the analyst will seek primarily psychodynamic balance (homeostasis), and therefore carefully avoid confronting the patient with the soul-searching quest for meaning and purpose. Frankl and his school, on the other hand, emphasize the relevance of the nöodynamic aspect and distinguish it from the psychodynamic. Psychodynamics cannot be sound and cannot lead towards health without the nöodynamic quest. In the normally sound and developing personality, there is always a wholesome gap between

the self and the self-ideal, between one's present existence and
one's aspirations. The healthy person accepts this nöodynamic
tension. On the other hand, 'too high a satisfaction with the self
indicates pathology.' [37]

Like humanistic trends in psychotherapy, logotherapy helps
the patient to a realistic awareness of the nöodynamic striving and
to an acceptance of this tension between realization and ideal
as a reminder of man's pilgrim situation. This therapeutic
approach, however, has nothing to do with an abominable
imperative moralism that would impose commandments and
precepts on a man without consideration for the *kairos* and without heeding his stage of development. Logotherapy gradually
leads a person to the consciousness of his own responsibility
according to the uniqueness of his personality and the singularity
of his situation. This process cannot even be initiated with an
arbitrary or one-sided voluntarism. Appeal to the will to search
for meaning implies a manifestation of meaning and purpose,
and a leaving it totally to the free will to decide for it subse-
quently.[38] Through this respectful orientation towards meaning
in a common search, the patient gradually becomes able to accept
his unique responsibility in relation to the world and to the
people about him. He will find his own self in the courage to
accept responsible relationships.

4. *Psychotherapy and secular pastoral care*

We have already indicated the dangers which lurk in
psychoanalysis when it tries to enlarge consciousness without
elevating it to the level of moral awareness in freedom and
responsibility. Psychoanalysis then remains indifferent to moral
values. Without the necessary distinctions, all feelings of guilt
and failure are explained in purely psychological terms as a
complex. With a certain irony, Gertrude von LeFort speaks of
'the absolution of the psychoanalyst who recognizes no sin which

---

[37] G.W. Allport, *Personality, op. cit.*, p. 161.
[38] V. Frankl, *Arztliche, op. cit.*, pp. 76-77.

cannot be forgiven because there is no freedom that can turn to God; and hence, the neurotic arrives at that awful liberation on which thousands thrive, whose illness, in last analysis, is nothing else than scorn for the peace of God.' [39]

In a very different direction, Viktor Frankl develops his idea of the secular doctor of the soul. He remains faithful to the best insights of psychotherapy, quite aware that the psychotherapist must begin by first liberating the unconscious, by releasing the psychic forces before freedom and responsibility can be summoned to a new response. How else would man find the full extent of his response-ability? The priest and the therapist should co-operate in this direction; each has his own *kairos*, his proper moment. But practically, so often in this age of secularization and because of new competences, the psychotherapist has replaced the pastor. The logotherapist shies away from an all too simplified psychoanalytic confession or absolution. His ministry is to heal the soul in a secularized world through his special competence and intimate personal relationship made possible through psychotherapeutic transference and companionship in the quest for meaning. The logotherapist, however, is not expected to replace religion and religious pastoral care.[40] His approach and techniques are grounded in the firm conviction of the uniqueness and absolute dignity of each person and man's vocation to search for the meaning of his life and accept his own responsibility. Such is the holistic concept of health encompassed by logotherapy.

What Frankl posits as principles for the secular doctor of the soul can also help the priest to learn absolute respect for the conscience of others. The competent psychotherapist will never try to impose his faith, ideology or *Weltanschauung* on his patient nor will he ever absolve him from his own responsibility. All that he can do is to help him find the uniqueness of his own personality, the singularity of each *kairos* with the courage to

[39] Gertrude von LeFort, *Das Schweisstuch der Veronika* (München, 1935), p. 349.
[40] Frankl, *Arztliche, op. cit.,* pp. 223-240.

search for the purpose of his life and to accept the challenge
that comes from it.

When the psychotherapist and patient have the same religious
faith the course of treatment and logotherapeutic dialogue will
differ from that in cases where they come from quite different
religions, ideologies or backgrounds. But in all situations,
absolute respect for the conscience of the patient is the decisive
condition for helping him find his own response-ability. The
gradualness and wisdom of the procedure arise from the
knowledge that responsibility has to grow from the depth of a
person's insight, conviction and conscience. The logotherapist
will respectfully search for the vital points of departure in the
patient himself, in order to free the longing for meaningfulness
from psychic blockages. In this respect, the therapist helps the
patient to find the meaning of his illness and particularly of his
neurosis, to accept what cannot be healed immediately in order
to set free all the energies for healing whatever can be healed,
and to exercise as fully as possible his freedom within its given
limitations.

Frankl is profoundly convinced that the believer sees meaning
in a more personalistic way if, behind the word of life, he finds
God, the One who calls him and invites him to transcend himself in response to him who is Word and Love, who calls together
all men to transcend themselves in unity and solidarity.[41] But
human health is in sight whenever man can transcend his ego
in search of truth and in a genuinely human relationship with
the Thou.

5. Psychiatry and moral problems

Psychotherapy and psychiatry pose innumerable, serious
moral questions. We can still subscribe to the moral principles
formulated some twenty years ago: 'There is no objection, on
principle and in general, to psychoanalysis or any other form of
psychotherapy. Psychiatrists, psychotherapists, however, must

---

[41] *Ibid.*, p. 73.

observe the cautions dictated by sound morality, such as: avoiding the error of pansexualism, never counselling even material sin, respecting secrets that the patient is not permitted to reveal, avoiding disproportionate risks of moral dangers.' [42] The expression 'never counselling even material sin' need not be pressed to the point of deterring a therapist from advising the patient to act according to his own conscience if it is erroneous. Of course, the therapist will not, of his own initiative, suggest some action which is in itself intrinsically evil if this does not spring from the patient's own conscience. However, as repeatedly emphasized, the psychotherapist does not moralize by an untimely insistence on moral duties which are here-and-now out of a patient's reach. Even the pastor will not insist on duty if he realizes that a person is still lacking the necessary insight and freedom. For example, the therapist will not speak of a moral obligation to avoid masturbation unless this is necessary now for progressive maturation. As long as his patient is not at the point of overcoming the problem and provided it does not stand as an obstacle to healing, the doctor will refrain from mentioning it or speaking as a 'moralist' if his patient refers to it.

The choice of a psychiatrist or psychotherapist is of utmost importance to a patient's future. For better or for worse, the therapist exercises a tremendous power over his patient's psychic life. Consequently, he can influence his moral attitudes and full range of social relationships. Relatives, friends or counsellors who recommend a psychiatrist must exercise great care and seek proper information. Responsibility in this field is even greater than in the choice of a doctor who treats organic illnesses.

What we have said earlier about the physician's duty to test all his procedures in the light of the history of freedom and liberation applies in a very particular way to the psychiatrist.

---

[42] *Ethical and Religious Directives for Hospitals* (2nd ed., 1955), No. 46. The 1971 revision of these directives makes no reference whatsoever to psychotherapeutic procedures; they seem to be subsumed under general therapeutic procedures in view of the total good of the patient.

The decisive criterion must be the hoped-for increase in genuinely human freedom. It belongs absolutely to the standards of good treatment that the therapist never become involved sexually with a patient. Such behaviour would violate even the most basic rules and prospects of genuine transference.

Moral theology is not competent to determine the cases in which certain procedures and methods are to be applied, but a doctor is duty-bound to proceed with absolute responsibility in full knowledge of the possible consequences. On principle, there is no objection to hypnotism or electroshock therapy if such methods are medically indicated.

The last decades have benefited by the discovery of an auxiliary procedure, narcoanalysis, for which criteria have gradually been elaborated in view of its proper application. The treatment consists of an intravenous administration of very refined dosages of barbiturates which place the patient in a semi-conscious state. The goal is to allow the subconscious to be unblocked more easily and to manifest its contents in the anamnesis. There are advantages despite the dangers inherent in the procedure. An undesirable repression is lifted in relation to the images mounting from the patient's subconscious and selective control over them is diminished; this might be an advantage. On the other hand, suggestibility by the therapist is heightened to the point that the patient's state sometimes borders on the hypnotic. If psychoanalysis has its many pitfalls owing to the conscious or subconscious influence of the therapist on the whole reaction of the patient, then *a fortiori*, there are greater dangers in the procedures of narcoanalysis. For this reason, exceptionally high professional and moral competence is demanded of the therapist who is convinced that narcoanalysis should be used at a certain point.

While I do not object to a moderate use of narcoanalysis by an experienced and responsible therapist who has the explicit or at least reasonably-presumed consent of the patient, use of the 'truth serum' as a medical procedure in court or police interrogations must be thoroughly rejected. It then becomes an infringement of freedom, a new method for extorting confessions, whether true or false. Finally, when 'truth drugs' are combined with other methods of brainwashing in a concerted effort to derange a human personality, the modern state has reached the culmination of inhumanity. No responsible doctor will cooperate in such an abuse.

Psychosurgery (for example lobotomy and leukotomy) is a relatively new surgical advance in psychiatry. It is founded on the supposition that certain psychic reactions can be localized in the brain. Consequently, serious behavioural disturbances can be eliminated or at least greatly reduced by the section of the thalamic frontal tracts. The operation was first performed in 1936 by De Martel and Moniz, and since then has been repeated thousands of times with varying degrees of success. Such a surgical procedure normally follows a very penetrating psycho-analytic treatment. The positive results of lobotomy enable the mentally ill to live a more agreeable and socially adjusted life, but secondarily, there is a visible restriction of personality in the sense of a diminution of motivation and energy for personal decision and initiative. It somehow alters a personality, but in severe cases of mental illness the lessened excitability far out-weighs the damage. 'Lobotomy and similar operations are morally justified when medically indicated in the proper treatment of serious mental illness or intractable pain. In each case the welfare of the patient himself, considered as a person, must be the determining factor. These operations are not justifiable when less extreme remedies are reasonably available or in cases in which the probability of harm to the patient outweighs the hope of benefit for him.' [48]

Most psychiatrists agree with these fundamental criteria which illumine cases in the whole field of psychiatry. Further progress in psychotherapeutics should lessen the need for pro-cedures as drastic as lobotomy. The older pre-frontal lobotomy

---

[48] *Ethical and Religious Directives for Hospitals, op. cit.,* No. 44. The 1971 revision of these directives does not specify applications of the general principle enunciated in its Article 26: 'Therapeutic procedures which are likely to be dangerous are morally justifiable for proportionate reasons.'

is already falling into disuse and is being replaced by refined neurosurgical techniques.

6. *Therapy: homosexuality and similar disturbances*

Homosexuality is here considered as one of the most common sexual aberrations. To some extent, the following discussion is also valid for other sexual deviations and perversions.

Earlier times simply classified the homosexual as a criminal; this resulted either in his being ostracized as a leper or subjected to the gravest of punishments. Owing to progress in medical science, genetics and psychology, we now find ourselves able to discriminate the psychological disturbance from a blend of sin and suffering. New diagnostic criteria permit easy identification, but in view of the burden of suffering and frustration borne by homosexuals, there is need for more systematic studies and research bearing on prophylaxis and therapy. Until now, most of the scientific efforts have focused on male homosexuality. This is justified in part because the problem among women (lesbianism) appears to be less widespread, and does not lead to the same social pathology as in the male.

(a) *Sex deviants differ*

Experts are most careful about labelling a person 'homosexual.' There are countless persons who are deeply troubled by the fear of being homosexual, and in certain countries, this phobic anxiety is widespread. Neurotics who are tormented by the fear of bearing the homosexual stigma become obsessively concerned and examine themselves interminably for telltale signs in their body or in their attitudes. The misgiving is often triggered by an imprudent remark on the part of a friend or relative.[44] In no way, however, does the phobia serve as a sound protection against homosexuality; the anxiety can actually lead to a mental or nervous collapse. Therefore, doctors and counsellors have to be

---

[44] A. Massone, *Cause e terapia dell'omosessualità* (Edizioni OARI, Varese, 1970), p. 83.

extremely cautious in their expressions, examinations and tests, so as not to arouse irrational fears.

For good reasons, scientists in different countries refuse to call 'homosexuals' persons who, in spite of their one-sided like-sex attraction, do not manifest overt homosexual behaviour. Many therefore propose a distinction between homosexuality and homo-philia, whereby the term *homosexuality* would be restricted to cases of long-standing overt sexual activity based on preferential tendencies for the subject's own sex, while *homophilia* would refer to cases where the tendencies are kept on the level of marginally erotic friendships free of indecent behaviour.

Sporadic homosexual acts during adolescence are not indi-cative of a homosexual heritage or tendency, nor do they, in most cases, lead to a like-sex fixation. Occasional acts of the kind are all too often founded on an unhealthy exploratory curiosity in reaction to over-suspicious controls. Even adults are known to indulge temporarily in homosexual activities when cut off from their usual heterosexual relationships; they return to 'normalcy' as soon as the usual conditions of their life are restored. The seduction of the young, however, can lead to homosexual fixation in cases of latent predisposition, especially if youngsters are frequently abused by persons on whom they depend educationally. It is precisely for this reason that most modern legislatures protect the young against corruption by adults through imposing severe sanctions on seducers. Since the percentage of latent homosexuals or of ambivalents is adjudged to be relatively high (some estimate about twenty per cent of males), it becomes evident that the protection of youth is mandatory. This high percentage of latency also attests to the influence of the environment on the plastic personality of youth.

In many instances, individuals manifest overt homosexual behaviour patterns despite a primarily heterosexual or at least ambivalent constitution. These cases can be rather easily resolved if the patient is eager to free himself and if the partners involved will grant him freedom. A happy marriage can then remedy the situation. Frequently, however, homosexual tendencies are combined with and linked to other psychopathologies and neuroses. Therapy must then be oriented towards the healing of the total personality, seeking a new balance within the dynamic components of the sexual deviant.

(b) *Is homosexuality an illness?*

A number of studies maintain that homosexuality, while not fitting into the sexual norm, eludes classification as illness.[45] From our holistic view of health, however, it is surely a dysfunction which calls pressingly for medical help. Any sexual aberration which does not allow a person to find fulfilment in married love or in a balanced life of celibacy proves to be a grave encumbrance to freedom and joy, and troublesome in interpersonal relationships. Of course, we have to be critically discerning of those cases in which a pseudo-homosexual indulges in homosexual activity, such as homosexual prostitution, for immoral motives, and this in spite of an inherited normal heterosexual constitution. Most cases encountered by physicians, however, are truly homosexuals who suffer deeply under this aberration.

From the viewpoint of both medical ethics and total health, we need to differentiate cases of homosexual behaviour where a genuine moral effort and a deepened conversion towards love of God and neighbour would suffice to overcome the difficulty, from the numerous others where medical and/or psychotherapeutic assistance is absolutely necessary. In my opinion, a statement that 'the homosexual, as well as the heterosexual, is able to exercise control over the expressions of his sexual instinct'[46] is an unjustified oversimplification of the problem. This can be true only in cases of relatively weak homosexual tendencies not weighed down by other psychopathologies. Persons who seek medical assistance in solving this problem generally admit being unable to control their impulsive sexual tendencies. Our basic principle

---

[45] A good review of the literature in support of this stance can be found in the article of John P. Rush, 'Reforming Pastoral Attitudes Toward Homosexuality,' *Union Seminary Quarterly Review*, XXV (1970), pp. 439-455.

[46] Michael J. Buckley, *Morality and Homosexuality* (London, 1959).

would be applicable here: the goal of medical assistance is to heal what can be healed, to help the patient bear what cannot be healed, and to search for the meaning of suffering and the means for transcending it. Unwarranted moralizing can be a grave injustice to persons incapable of controlling their homosexual urge despite a sincere desire to do so.

(c) *Therapy*

A great number of authoritative reports reflect a pessimistic outlook on the prospect of healing the typical homosexual. It follows, then, that much more has to be done in terms of prophylaxis because of the sociopathological causes and implications of homosexuality. More is mandatory also in the field of individual therapy. With progress in diagnosis and in the differentiation of sexual anomalies, the possibilities of healing are constantly enhanced. Genetic studies have contributed valuable insights into the determination of genotypical sex through a study of chromosomes.[47] The hereditary character seems incontrovertible in many instances.[48] There are cases of anomalous sexual differentiation and others which are related to constitutional variants or inadequacies.[49] But most studies concur that the majority of homosexual problems are either caused or at least aggravated by erratic behaviour patterns in the familial or immediate social environment.

It is only in the last few decades that psychoanalysis and psychotherapy have progressed substantially in anamnesis and hence in the treatment of homosexuals who are victims of parental inadequacies and conflicts. Only a long-lasting depth therapy can help the afflicted since the whole of the personality suffers from the consequences of countless repressions.[50] Most homosexuals reported deeply disturbed parent-child relationships; the parents

---

[47] A. Massone, *Cause e terapia, op. cit.*, pp. 112 ff.
[48] *Ibid.*, pp. 117-118.
[49] *Ibid.*, p. 133.
[50] Cf.: Irving Bieber, *Homosexuality. A Psychoanalytic Study of Male Homosexuals* (New York: Basic Books, 1963).

were found to have had grave emotional problems. The child then bore the burden of parental conflicts.[51] Bieber's study proves that patients who are really troubled by their homosexual leanings and want to be healed can be helped, but there is need of depth therapy.

Not all cases of homosexuality are equally affected by the structure of parent-child relationships; some prove more amenable to cure than others. The present development points towards the need for multifaceted approaches and methods. So far, hormonal treatment has proved ineffective since it only heightened the sexual desire.[52] Without a complete psychoanalysis, a number of patients can be helped through simpler anamnetic methods to the point where the overt homosexuality is reduced to a latent form with the capacity for heterosexual relationships. To transform an overt homosexual into a latent one truly represents a therapeutic success.[53] This point has to be stressed particularly in view of the fact that for most of the patients, complete psychoanalytic treatment is not yet available, either for lack of competent therapists or for lack of financial means.

In some cultures, homosexuality springs not so much from faulty parent-child relationships as from an inadequate or warped sexual education which mainly presents the opposite sex as dangerous. Defensive reactions against the other sex crystallize into a firm ego-protective system and attention is superficially turned to like-sexed partners. There are effective therapeutic means, including anamnesis, that can uncover and help overcome this distortion.

With respect to disorders emerging from a patient's newly-found relationships with persons of the opposite sex, the

---

[51] Edeltrud Meistermann-Seeger, in Michael Buckley, *Morality and Homosexuality, op. cit.,* Postscript, p. 220.

[52] Cf.: Jacques Decourt and Paul Guinet, *Les états intersexuels* (Paris: Librairie Maloine, 1962). The authors' conclusion that psychoanalysis alone can help is being abandoned more and more.

[53] A. Massone, *Cause e terapia, op. cit.,* p. 197.

therapist will never encourage whatever is against the principles of morality, but neither will he obstruct the process of healthy transformation by an excessive moralism which would practically repeat the earlier pedagogical error of the parents. Logotherapy would seem indicated for such cases. The patient should be helped to find the meaning of sexuality and of the conjugal-parental vocation if he is to find fulfilment in genuine married love. It is of paramount importance to cast the process of change in the light of the morality of growth and of continual conversion; to adhere to a static view of abstract principles can be most damaging.

7. The therapy of drug addition and alcoholism

All that we have said relative to a concept of total human health, with particular emphasis on the development of human freedom, comes to a juncture in the matter of drug addiction. It could well be that no other problem transcends so totally the limits of a purely individualistic, merely somatic and barely therapeutic vision seeking symptomatic relief. The problem of drug addiction and alcoholism forces us to a comprehensive study of the biography, the ecology and total situation of the patient. Today the problem has reached proportions which compel the whole of society, especially the medical profession, to research into its manifold interwoven causes and to trace a holistic course for its prevention and healing.

Drug addiction and alcoholism have always called for a multidimensional therapy; they can be considered together as basically similar social and psychological problems.[54] Besides the personal psychosomatic aspect, the patient's family or immediate environment enter the picture as far as treatment is concerned. Because of its rapidly increasing incidence among young people today, drug abuse is particularly serious as a worldwide social problem. Alcoholism exists more commonly among adults, and in some countries it is still on the increase. Owing however to

---

[54] World Health Organization Technical Report Series, (1967), No. 363.

its intrinsic part in the recreations of adult life in western culture, society more readily tolerates deviant behaviour associated with alcohol than deviant behaviour associated with drugs such as marijuana, heroin and LSD.[55] It remains that alcoholism is similar to drug addiction in its etiology and results.

(a) The various forms of addiction

The immense cost to humanity of widespread drug addiction is well documented historically. The opium wars of Great Britain against China, which led to the opium addiction of at least twenty to thirty million Chinese and many other oriental people, constitute one of the most shocking situations in modern history. Probably more than anything else, the lethargy arising from the use of opium accounts for the social underdevelopment of China and could be one of the main causes for the victory of communism there. Cannabis (marijuana) and other intoxicating herbs brought the millions of South American Indians to their apathy and inactivity, without which the actual underdevelopment of Latin America would be inexplicable. The situation is similar in many Arab countries, in Afghanistan for instance, where hashish is widely used.

Alcohol, nicotine and caffeine are usually considered domestic drugs. The most widespread of all addictions and one of the main causes of lung cancer is the addiction to excessive smoking. Abuse of nicotine not only shortens a man's life expectancy but results in a typical loss of freedom and energy. The psychologically less damaging caffeine and nicotine addictions however, do not reveal the same adverse effects on the whole personality structure as do alcohol, heroin and LSD.

Alcohol, which used to be the drug of the poor and desperate, has become an integral part of the unending-pleasure-seeking individuals who lead an unfulfilled life in our wealthy society. Of course, one needs to distinguish an occasional abuse of alcohol in any of its various forms from addiction to it.

---

[55] Gordon Claridge, *Drugs and Human Behaviour* (London: Penguin Press, 1970), p. 224.

Drugs associated with addiction are generally classified as sedative, stimulant or hallucinogenic. Stimulant drugs taken for alertness during examinations and other similar occasions do not generally lead to dependency although they could. Today the socio-pathological drug scene is focused primarily on the 'hard drugs' like the opiates, morphine, heroin and cocaine, which lead to the heaviest form of addiction and loss of freedom, to criminality, and finally to severe brain damage. Besides these, there are numberless drugs considered to be potentially habit-forming, such as the barbiturates and amphetamines, cannabis (marijuana) and some of the hallucinogenic compounds. In the hands of responsible doctors and psychiatrists, many drugs serve a healing purpose, but they should be used only under controlled conditions and in controlled quantities since the danger of addiction lurks even there. In some countries, lack of protection against abuse of the multitudinous existing medications is a particularly grave problem.

(b) *Crime or sickness?*

The black market in drugs is undoubtedly one of the most criminal situations today. Running up and down the whole gamut from the ever-rising spread of marijuana and hashish to the encouragement of opium, morphine, heroin and cocaine, criminal organizations bring diverse pressure tactics to bear on the sick, who would like to liberate themselves from enslavement to drugs but are unable to do so by themselves. The threat of denunciation to legal authorities often deters an addict from seeking help, and all too often, even the parents of addicts dare not bring their children to the physician because of the fear of having them denounced as criminals.

We should consider drug addicts as fundamentally sick persons, and addiction as an illness to which society, and specifically the medically competent, should respond. In no way does this attitude absolve the addicts of their share of moral responsibility for their actual situation. Whatever therapy is initiated has to appeal to their still existing though limited freedom, but without any judgmental attitude on the part of the therapist.

N

The vocation of the doctor is to heal and not to sit in judgment on others. He is expected to search for the causes of a patient's distress and accordingly to prescribe the most appropriate and effective remedy.

The question of whether addiction is 'crime' or 'sickness' takes on new significance in view of today's worldwide phenomenon of drug abuse among the young. Legislation and public opinion should not equate experimentation with or abuse of marijuana, hashish and psychedelics with experimentation with, or abuse of the most dangerous drugs like morphine and heroin. Confusion of this type becomes especially irritating when the most vocal censors of the 'drug culture' are more (certainly not less) addicted to alcohol and smoking, but they do not dream of putting themselves in the category of 'addicts'. I am not implying that we should minimize the harmful effects of these lesser drugs or that we should be indifferent to protective legislation against them. The young need to be properly informed and insofar as possible protected, but there is little hope of persuading them if adult judgment is warped or lacking in a sense of distinction.

Today's youth levels accusations of pharisaism against a society which evades its own responsibility while severely punishing sick drug addicts whose illness arises in a considerable measure from social disorders. It is a pitiful phenomenon that our society is neither ready nor willing to examine its structures, customs, philosophies, behaviour and prejudices which trigger the downfall of so many people into crime, or so-called crime, which realistically is better termed sickness.

(c) *The main causes of the actual situation in drug addiction*

The particular causes of addiction in an individual case must be clearly distinguished from the social causes of such a widespread disorder as the present addiction of the young and of a great many adults. Serious investigators agree on the general factors leading to dependency on drugs: (1) the availability of drugs, (2) the exent to which a community or subculture accepts a drug as socially harmless, and (3) the extent of exposure to different drugs. Given availability, the extent of exposure becomes for the individual consumer an important factor in the pattern of addiction.[56]

Social pressures for conformity lead many teen-agers to experiment with drugs, with the inherent danger of promotion to 'harder' drugs. This point of view is substantiated by evidence 'that almost all heroin addicts, for example, have graduated to narcotics from other drugs like amphetamines and cannabis.' [57] There is speculation that the risk may be a social rather than a pharmacological one, but not enough evidence has yet been gathered on the escalation or long-range effects to form a sound judgment. In any event, 'once having made contact with the drug-taking subcultures in society, the individual finds himself increasingly caught up in their web and tempted to seek the new excitement of more powerfully addictive drugs.' [58]

While the immediate causes of individual dependency on drugs are multiple, the accusing finger points to the person's social environment. Personal reasons can range from a single traumatic event to a confused and troubled background, marital or familial conflicts, feelings of insecurity, and anxiety. 'Among the young, the affluent and the bored, the road to habitual drug-taking may start with the desire for an "arousal jag" which stimulants like the amphetamines can offer. For the very anxious, it may begin with the discovery that barbiturates or alcohol enable them to cope with social situations that would otherwise be agony to bear. Those who go on to swell the ranks of the "hard" drug addicts may have severe personality problems traceable to a variety of events in their life histories.' [59]

An example from a quite different field may illustrate this difference between personal and social causation. If the Breton who lives in a totally Catholic area does not participate in the life of the Church, his reasons are very personal — perhaps an unsanctioned marriage or a quarrel with the local priest; but the

---

[56] *Ibid.*, p. 226.
[57] *Ibid.*, p. 228.
[58] *Ibid.*, p. 228.
[59] *Ibid.*, p. 229.

fact that a high percentage of migrant workers coming from Brittany to dechristanized areas give up participation in church life has to be explained mainly by environmental causes. Similarly, numerous cases of alcoholism and drug addiction can be explained by the biography of the person or by a particular pathology of a smaller bohemian group like artists, or by the 'contagion' of a certain milieu. There exists also a widespread problem of alcoholism as an expression of social destitution and despair under the pressures of dehumanizing life conditions: poor housing, joblessness, social contempt, and the like. The tranquilizing effects of escape are sought through drinking or through drugs if the environment so invites. Disorders against morals, health and the law are the result. Many psychologists, anthropologists and physicians have begun research into the etiology of such social pathology, and the corrective measures to be initiated or instituted.

In spite of the fact that personality-wise no 'addict type' has been clearly delineated, there are certain features common to all. Chronic alcoholics and confirmed narcotic addicts are generally described as immature and excessively dependent individuals, often sexually inadequate and having a history of poor interpersonal relationships. Drugs or alcohol enable them to deal with their personal deficiencies by escape into a make-believe world. The experienced 'high' enables them to adjust temporarily to the life stress that would otherwise threaten personality disintegration.[60] Peter Laurie's recent book on addiction discusses at length this point of view.[61]

I return once more to the problem of a collective nöogenic neurosis. In my opinion, the problem of the 'hippies' and the mass drug addiction of youth cannot be explained without an understanding of this neurosis pervading the whole environment and finding expression in aimlessness and meaninglessness in the midst of economic success and a comfortable life. Children are gorged with material possessions but are wanting in genuine

---

[60] *Ibid.*, pp. 229-230.
[61] Peter Laurie, *Drugs* (London: Penguin Press, 1967).

love and challenging ideals. In the young's reaction to empty materialism, there is discernible a healthy yearning for meaning and for commitment to a fully human life, but as they are somewhat contaminated by the collective neurosis, their reactions cannot be healthy in all manners and modes.

I also view the drug phenomenon as a symbol of protest against the 'establishment,' that economic, social, academic, political and religious conglomerate which, through impersonal and depersonalizing administration, is threatening what Camus has called 'that part of man which must always be defended.' Let us be mindful that youth's first protest was not by drugs. Led by the best of its generation, it was a valiant effort filled with the hope that the situation could be changed. The relative immobilism of the establishment strengthened and broadened the base of protest, but when change was not forthcoming, drugs came to the fore and expressed the dissent of the tired and disenchanted, who came from family environments marked by the same collective neurosis. They had neither the courage nor the endurance of those from healthier backgrounds who have continued the search for constructive ways of inducing change.

While individual causes of 'hippiedom' vary, flight into these subculture groups is often as much a mark of discouragement as of lack of fortitude. The disheartened want to 'stop the world and get off.' Their psychic energy drained, they no longer have the strength to continue their search for truth, meaning and commitment; in the midst of their conflict, they escape into the illusory make-believe drug world. Some still aim for deeper experiences, and so they try psychedelic drugs to enter the quasi-mystical environment and to share in pseudo-religious happenings. Their hopes are expressed in a language which is as unreal as that of the nöogenic neurosis and concomitant eccentricities which they are combating. They have not escaped the vicious circle; they have only reversed it.

Many parents of today's youth have not dared refuse anything to their children. To a considerable extent, parents and children alike have been victims of an overblown psychology of permissiveness which warned against the dangers of frustrating the child but not against the worse dangers of failing to develop his dynamism and integrative power through the growth-qualities of hope, will, purpose, competence. . . .[62] A youth-worshipping society wanted 'happiness' for the young, but the prevailing materialistic values and pleasure-seeking philosophy chose to give them a surfeit of 'things' rather than the self-giving love they craved for. Neither the home environment nor the school or community milieu opened them to steadfast values, setting them on the path to fulfilment, namely, that of commitment to ideals and significant work.

Long years of economic dependence, the nihilistic philosophy and literature to which many of the young are academically subjected, the constant barrage of violent and scandalous headlines to the exclusion of the good news ignored by the communications media, the claustrophobic conditions of urban life: all these ingredients of the mass nöogenic neurosis have contributed to the pattern of ego-failure among those who escape into groups of hippies for community and love without knowing yet what true community and true love mean.

That a great part of modern youth has lost the capacity to suffer, and to dedicate itself with endurance to a great goal comes very often from its having failed to grasp the meaning of life. In the same context, we need to consider the tremendous propensity of modern man to conformity. Youth looks at the world of adults with its smoking-drinking habits and levels the charge of *hypocrites* at those who condemn the new habits of young people while conforming to their old ones. Therefore, the attempts to resolve such a mass problem by suppression alone will only give new impetus to the escapist form of protest. Imposition of any directive from 'above' becomes a matter of discouragement and of juvenile obstinacy; yet youth is longing for a meaningful life.

---

[62] I use here Erik Erikson's titles for those 'virtues' which, in childhood, become the basis of ego-strength. See his chapter on 'Human Strength and the Cycle of Generations,' *Insight and Responsibility, op. cit.,* pp. 109-157.

If religion often fails to appeal to the younger generation, it is because of its one-sided conceptualization and juridical approach to orthodoxy, cult and life. Doctrinal teaching, the administration of the sacraments and even the liturgy tend to be all too cerebral. The insistence on uniform or stereotyped forms of worship does not penetrate the creative imagination of the young nor align with their idealism. Youth therefore is attracted to the magical 'liturgy' in which the psychedelic drug is celebrated. I feel strongly about the imperative need for further studies on this particular problem of the estrangement of our young people from religion. If we were able to instil into them faith in all its depth and to synthesize it with life, if we were zealous enough in presenting to them an attractive ideal truthfully, the mass phenomenon of youthful drug addiction would disappear or would at least be reduced to the marginal group of abnormals.[63]

(d) *Therapy*

In the more serious cases of addiction, particularly in the case of users of 'hard' drugs, persuasion alone will not suffice; physiological detoxification is called for. Unfortunately, psychological detoxification does not always follow. Pharmacological and psychological methods are constantly evolving and the physician needs to keep abreast of developments.

For persons who are really addicted to nicotine or alcohol, but not to drugs, healing becomes possible only if the patient accepts total abstinence; an occasional lapse into the old habit only serves to reactivate it. This is all the more so in the case of narcomania; the craving for the drug remains after the body has been detoxified, especially if psychotherapy has not succeeded in lifting the psychological dependency. In most cases of narcomania, hospitalization is absolutely necessary to initiate therapy. It would seem very important to give patients an opportunity for continued education during the long period of hospitalization.

---

[63] Giacomo Perico, 'Giovani e allucinogeni,' *Civiltà Cattolica*, 121 (1970), 417-433.

It is not unsusual for the social worker or consultant to contact the family since they too may need careful re-education, perhaps in the form of group therapy. Psychoanalysis takes a long time and it will not be effective without the patient's insertion into a healthier environment.

The experiences of Alcoholics Anonymous are very illuminating. Their success is based on a kind of in-group therapy, a good example of which can be seen in the 'guest house' erected near Detroit for the rehabilitation of alcoholic and drug-addicted clergymen. Their success rate is in the vicinity of eighty-five per cent. It is accounted for in part by the close teamwork of neurologist, psychologist and pastor, but hinges mostly on group therapy. There exists here a community founded on mutual respect and trust. Similar results, even with people far less motivated, are obtained in a number of communities organized by rehabilitated drug addicts.[64]

The healing process must gradually phase the rehabilitated addict back into society. There is still a problem relative to reinstating him in his family, in the labour force and in society at large. Here I return to the basic thesis: the whole of society or the particular environment of this person is sick. Prophylactic measures and constructive approaches are absolutely necessary. It may be that this is precisely the lesson God wants to teach us through the mass phenomenon of addiction.

C. *Various ethical issues in therapy*

A physician's ethical response in all professional activities is necessarily coloured by the depth and breadth of his concept of health and therapy. Morality is never a watertight compartment cut off from life; rather, it represents the whole meaning of human activity and relationship. Such is the framework

---

[64] Cf.: J. Durand-Dassier, *Psychothérapies sans psychothérapeute.* Communauté de drogués et de psychotiques (Paris, 1970). Reference to Daytop explains one rehabilitative approach to drug addiction.

within which a number of therapeutic questions will now be discussed.

Our attention turns first to the physician-patient relationship with regard to fostering an atmosphere of truthfulness and trust especially in observing confidentiality, in taking responsibility for imparting information to the patient about the prospects and risks of the therapeutic methods adopted, and the monetary expenses involved. Special consideration must be given to the patient's personality prior to undertaking treatments likely to cause moral difficulties for him, for example, the risk of drug addiction. Plastic surgery and painless childbirth will be mentioned as two different but typical examples of how the doctor has to assess the overall effects of his medical action with respect to the patient's personal life. The specifically human point of view becomes especially crucial when the dearth of personnel, facilities or equipment for a life-saving procedure necessitates the doctor's choosing among several patients.

1. *The physician-patient relationship*

Ramsey gives to his book on ethical problems in medicine the significant title, *The Patient as Person*.[65] He thus pinpoints accurately the central concept and main criterion for a wholesome physician-patient relationship in so far as it influences or conditions the patient's outlook and response to medical therapy. The ethos of the doctor, as well as his whole approach to effective treatment, depends considerably on an optimal interpersonal relationship between physician and patient.

The doctor-patient tie is a covenant of persons. In times of serious illness and in the total ordering of the medical profession, the contribution of the doctor can never be severed from personal concern. The privacy and intimate reactions of the ailing person transcend by far the impersonal basis of many other relationships. While the seller-buyer contract is founded on commutative

---

[65] Paul Ramsey, *The Patient as Person* (New Haven: Yale University Press, 1970).

justice, the relationship between doctor and patient is distinguished and characterized by such personal attitudes as fidelity, reverence, respect, truthfulness and mutual trust. If the doctor wants to do justice to the patient by caring for his total health and helping him to accept his illness and discover its personal meaning, he must regard the sick human being in his uniqueness, with inviolable personal rights and expectations. He must also take into account the patient's relationship to God, his fellowmen and society, particularly his family.

A physician's fidelity and responsibility towards his patient entail a correlative responsibility towards his fellowmen and society, although it is not always simple to reconcile the interests of the patient with those of society. At times the dilemma of medical ethics seems insoluble because of the need to consider the patient on the one hand, as a distinct individual, and on the other, as a constituent member of a society which sets claims upon him. The physician's resolution not to depart from the concept of the patient as a person is decisive ethically; such a stance necessarily includes his essential relationships and responsibilities to his fellowmen. In this frame of reference, the doctor does not violate the fidelity of his covenant if he fails to accede to a patient's selfish and irresponsible wishes but acts according to the best interests and personal calling of the patient. In grave cases, after having exhausted all means of persuading a patient to responsible action, the physician may be compelled to protect the just expectations and rights of his fellow-citizens and of society even against the patient's will.

I have already mentioned the importance of an atmosphere of truthfulness and trust in the crucial matter of the doctor's deportment when faced by the prospect of a patient's death. Only if we understand fully the import of these qualities in the covenant between physician and patient can we realize the attitude proper to a doctor as death approaches. On the other hand, we have also seen how a guarded truthfulness in this extreme situation influences the patient-physician relationship in the matter of therapy. Truthfulness and trust from both patient and doctor are needed, but it is chiefly the veracity and trustworthiness of the physician that condition responsiveness and confidence in the patient.

2. *Professional secrecy*

The significance of the covenant of trust linking doctor and patient becomes most critical in the matter of confidentiality. Professional secrecy is an essential component of the medical ethos. The oath of Hippocrates says: 'If it be what should not be noised abroad I will keep silence thereon.' The American Medical Association code declares: 'Confidence ... should never be revealed unless the law requires it or it is necessary to protect the welfare of individuals or communities.'

In almost all countries, the law requires that contagious diseases be reported. Such a request is absolutely justified by the common good in spite of the fact that it may be most unpleasant for the diseased person. Beyond the legal obligation and on the grounds of his medical ethos, the doctor will evince concern that other persons be not unnecessarily exposed to the danger of contagion. Even in highly developed countries, the general population is not yet sufficiently protected against contamination by communicable diseases, open tuberculosis for instance. The immediate family should be informed of proper methods of protecting itself and friends. Care should be taken that contagious persons do not use any public facilities as long as they constitute a considerable threat as 'carriers'.[66]

It is first of all the patient's obligation to show responsibility towards the people with whom he lives. The doctor or, where available, the social worker or member of the community medical team, ought to explain to him the situation and the consequences of irresponsible behaviour. The adult patient should then be expected to act responsibly, but if he cannot, or if he proves unwilling to do so, the physician must assume his part of the

---

[66] R. Arnoldt, 'Seuchenhygienisch bedenkliche Verschwiegenheit bei ansteckungsfähiger Lungentuberkulose,' *Praxis der Pneumologie*, 22 (1968), 176-182.

responsibility in keeping with the principle of subsidiarity, so as to protect the patient and society.[67]

In cases where the physician cannot motivate or convince the patient of his duty to communicate what he should, the doctor himself becomes accountable. But before informing others, because of special responsibilities, the doctor has to ponder well all the values at stake. There are situations, for example, in cases of venereal disease, when even though others may be exposed to some danger or damage, it may be better to keep silent than to make use of information which has been obtained professionally, with the inevitable risk of diminishing the patient's trust. It is not just the relationship of this one patient to this one doctor that is in jeopardy. One doctor's imprudent use of confidence, should it come to the knowledge of others, can impair the relationship of many doctors with their patients. Only when there is serious danger for others is the doctor allowed or obliged to speak when a patient refuses to fulfil an obvious obligation to make known his infectious disease.

Every patient should be aware that when he reveals his condition to a physician, the doctor can never be a willing accomplice to crime by an unjustified silence. Secrecy can never become a taboo. Observance or non-observance must always be judged with respect to the welfare of the patient and of all other persons involved. The saying, 'The sabbath was made for man and not man for the sabbath' applies also to secrecy.

The physician's obligation to secrecy is protected and sanctioned by most legislatures. In court a doctor can, on general principle, reveal confidential information only if the patient has agreed to waive his right to confidentiality. The psychotherapist-patient right to privileged communication should be absolute before any court. The psychotherapist must never, before a tribunal or others, make use of any confidential material that could be prejudicial to his patient, even if the patient has expli-

---

[67] Cf.: Henry A. Davidson, 'Professional Secrecy,' in *Ethical Issues in Medicine,* ed. E.F. Torrey (Boston: Little, Brown and Co., 1968), p. 193.

citly waived the right of confidentiality. The reasons seem to me convincing: (a) the relationship between the therapist and patient demands an unusual amount of trust and therefore, of secrecy; (b) 'the psychiatrist, almost without exception, has no pertinent information. What he has is what he has been told by his patient: a collection of notions, feelings and sensations which, because of their highly subjective nature, may or may not have much in common with the kind of objective reality sought in the law court.' [68] No waiver should be acknowledged when the patient, because of his mental condition, does not have the necessary information and cannot estimate all the consequences of a waiver.

For the benefit of his patient or if necessary for the well-being of other persons, however, the therapist can and must sometimes speak with those to whom his patient is entrusted. For example, he may not only inform the spouse of a mentally disturbed patient that it is best to bear with him in the hope of improvement, but he may also discuss whether or not it is significant and possible, without grave dangers for the family, to continue living with him. The therapist may also deem it advisable to talk over with the spouse the prospect of continuance of the marriage.

3. *Informing the patient responsibly*

A trust-inspiring relationship between physician and patient demands, according to the situation, reliable information relative to the extent of risk attendant on certain treatments to be taken by the patient. It is understood that the doctor will first decide which treatment is most suitable so that he will not propose indifferently a number of possibilities which the patient himself would have to examine in order to find out which would best serve him. In most cases, it is incumbent on the physician to decide on the desirability of a treatment, but whenever a certain

---

[68] Paul F. Slawson, 'Patient-Litigant Exception,' *Archives of General Psychiatry,* 21 (September, 1969), 351-352.

procedure or operation entails considerable risk, he will inform the patient adequately in view of the total situation of his health. Were the disclosure of such information to constitute a risk of grave harm to the patient, the doctor will renounce doing it directly. Instead he may choose to inform members of the family and await the final decision from them.

The physician will refrain from using new and yet unproved medication or therapeutic means when a better or equally good prospect with lesser risk is available. Similarly, the doctor will not prefer a very expensive treatment to a relatively less expensive one if both serve the same purpose unless the patient or his family, after accurate information, explicitly indicate preference for the more costly method. Whenever there is question of using very expensive treatments with no real prospect of success, the physician should not burden the patient or his family with a decision since they would not enjoy the full freedom of spirit to say 'no' although they might be resentful of the idea. He should unilaterally decide to renounce such a course of action; it would be against the physician-patient covenant to impose on the patient's family extremely high expenses for a treatment which holds no promise of substantial help.

4. *Treatment constituting potential moral risk for the patient*

The physician's responsibility is particularly great when he resorts to medication or treatment which can cause moral danger to the patient. The concept of full human health serving as a basis for ethical considerations obliges him to include in his diagnostic efforts all the elements of his patient's particular endowment and character, such as for instance, *abulia* or weakness of the will. He may have to renounce hormonal treatments which can stimulate sexual desire beyond the patient's capacity for self-control.

Should a therapist consider hypnosis as a part of treatment, he has then to inform the patient honestly and seek his permission. No one ever entrusts himself so totally to possible manipulation by a therapist without making an explicit judgment that the therapist is worthy of this great moral trust. The therapist must also ask himself whether such a procedure will truly serve his patient in terms of promoting his moral freedom.

Particular caution is to be exercised in the use of sedatives and other drugs likely to constitute for certain individual patients a danger of addiction. Especially serious in consequence would be to risk such treatment when a patient has previously manifested a propensity towards drug addiction.

The hormonal control of pregnancy in the case of unmarried women, especially of young girls, poses serious moral problems for the doctor. He can often foresee that his prescription will be a further step towards moral laxity. On the other hand, his refusal to prescribe may well result in an abortion in the case of an undesired pregnancy. His decision needs serious reflection. If by medical arguments he cannot change the patient's attitude, then a realistic approach may avoid the greater danger. Where law makes the permission of the parents mandatory, the doctor will not resort to any subterfuge. Even where there is no legal interdiction to the treatment of a minor without parental permission, the doctor will not forget his responsibility towards the family. He will consult the parents to the extent he can without abdicating his own responsibility.

5. Painless childbirth

The pangs of childbirth are reckoned among the strongest pains experienced by human beings. This is so especially if there is great apprehension, as in cases of women who either have not fully and gladly accepted the pregnancy or have been frightened by over-anxious friends or, indeed, are so totally uninformed that they do not know what to expect.

In recent years, medicine and psychology have combined efforts in developing several methods of 'painless' childbirth. More and more the pregnant woman goes regularly, on a monthly or bimonthly basis, to her obstetrician for ample preparation. This offers a unique opportunity for the doctor to establish that covenant of trust and respect that helps him inspire confidence in the expectant mother. He will give her all the information that will help her to overcome anxiety and to look forward to the birth of her child. An appropriate and timely preparation for painless childbirth, especially through autogenetic training, increases the likelihood that the mother will experience the great moment of giving birth in full consciousness and joy.

Should the father wish to be with his wife at this moment, and if he can truly give moral support, trust and peace to her, the physician ought to accede to his request and prepare him accordingly. It will deepen his life as a person, and both father and mother can thus experience together the great family event. Methods which deprive the mother of full awareness at childbirth could well be eliminated today when other methods which allow consciousness are available.

6. Plastic (cosmetic) surgery

We are indebted to psychology for exposing the extent to which bodily blemishes can adversely affect a person's whole spiritual and psychological development. In fact, the body constitutes an essential component of the all-important self-concept.

Certain physical defects may be profoundly prejudicial to professional advancement and even to chances of marriage. They could thus jeopardize a conjugal and parental vocation for which someone would, otherwise, be well qualified. The physician therefore has a serious obligation to inform a child's parents that a birthmark or other superficial physical defect should be removed or corrected in due time by a harmless surgical procedure. If this is performed at an early age, success can usually be ensured with a minimum of discomfort for the child. On the other hand, a seriously intentioned surgeon does not lend his skill to certain types of plastic surgery meant only to satisfy a disturbed vanity or to cater to lower motives.

7. Who shall have priority for treatment?

Even in highly technically-developed countries, a dilemma of choice can be posed by the scarcity of medical resources. In my experience as medical assistant in an infantry regiment, it happened repeatedly that calls for help came simultaneously from injured men around me. I was once confronted with five seriously wounded soldiers, all of whom needed immediate attention. I could only help one after the other, and when I came to the last he was almost exsanguinated. A similar situation, though normally less dramatic, often confronts today's physician even in times of peace.

A serious question of conscience arises for the whole welfare society when there are not enough beds, equipment and personnel available in hospitals to serve patients in need of immediate assistance. Many trends have aggravated the situation in the course of the last several years. Shorter working hours for personnel were inaugurated at the very time when medical care and hospitalization were becoming available to more people than ever before. Concurrently, medical science and technology were (and still are) discovering new medication and techniques and inventing new life-saving machines. A considerable lag between discovery or invention and adequate production and implementation is unavoidable. Because of the scarcity of dialyzers, for example, many patients who otherwise could be saved are of necessity excluded from treatment. Such a problem is understandable in the initial phases of new medical advances, but once a technique has proved its worth, the whole medical profession and all influential citizens should join forces to remedy the situation as soon as possible. Today, hemodialysis treatment is not much more costly than was once the prolonged stay of a tubercular patient in a sanatorium.

Wherever a serious shortage of apparatus or of trained personnel makes it impossible to assist the whole pool of patients, the criteria for patient selection have to be determined from the medical standpoint in a truly professional and personalistic perspective. The decisive factor should be the probability of lasting success. It is immoral to monopolize apparatus for a few hours' prolongation of the life of a well-paying 'Very Important Person' when this robs of his chance a less wealthy person whose life could be saved for his family and for the service of society.

o

In the present capitalistic society, the individual physician will often be confronted with crucial decisions which place poorer patients in an unfavourable position. The common efforts of the medical profession, social reform and enlightened legislation should absolutely rule out the possibility of lower social classes not receiving necessary life-saving assistance while wealthier classes have at their disposal everything to prolong the dying process for days and weeks. A comprehensive survey conducted in the United States relative to 'Who is preferred' when there is an insufficient number of dialyzers shows that in most hospitals the decisive criterion was the greater medical suitability, the genuine chances of a lasting success. Further, a psychiatric consultation assessed the potential for vocational rehabilitation and the need for the patient to support his family. The statistics did reveal, however, that coloured people and the lower social classes were at a serious disadvantage.

D. *Experimentation with human beings*

Human life unfolds and attains increasingly higher levels through a developing process of experimentation which follows the long history of groping of the material and biological animal world. Without such groping and experimentation our existence in the present order of creation would be inconceivable. The progress of medicine, with its manifold benefits for mankind, owes a heavy debt to experimentation and research. Evidently, not all investigations further progress. The culturally responsive and responsible element of human society became acutely aware of this during the Nuremberg trials of physicians who had co-

---

[69] Albert H. Katz and Donald M. Procter, *Social-Psychological Characteristics of Patients Receiving Hemodialysis Treatment for Chronic Renal Failure*. Kidney Disease Programme, U.S. Department of Health, Education and Welfare, Contract No. PH 108-66-95, (July, 1969).
Cf.: comments of Paul Ramsey, *The Patient as Person, op. cit.*, p. 250.

operated with the Nazi government in experimentation with political prisoners, mentally retarded persons and members of other racial groups. It was a case of human persons being used ruthlessly as tools for investigation. Although scientific data may have been gathered, inhumane procedures and impersonal attitudes sketched a radical picture of decay and destruction of the medical ethos.

1. *The medical code on experimentation*

On the occasion of the Nuremberg process, a medical code was established as a basis for prosecuting scientists or researchers who experimented criminally with human beings.[70] This code has received considerable attention in professional literature.

Ethical codes and legislation governing medical practice express the ethical convictions of a society. It must be acknowledged that the Nuremberg Code on 'Permissible Medical Experiments' denotes a high professional ethos, possibly too stringent for its particular scope, that is, as a basis for grave sanctions. Under the impact of the horrifying events disclosed at the Nuremberg trials, the medical profession has continued to sharpen its conscience and to serve as a beacon for the whole world. A mature codification resulted in the *Declaration of Helsinki:* Recommendations Guiding Doctors in Clinical Research, a resolution adopted at the eighteenth World Medical Assembly in June of 1964 by the World Medical Association. Its soundness compels me to give here the full text:

THE DECLARATION OF HELSINKI

INTRODUCTION

It is the mission of the doctor to safeguard the health of the people. His knowledge and conscience are dedicated to the fulfilment of this mission.

---

[70] *Trials of War Criminals Before the Nuremberg Military Tribunals Under Control Council Law No. 10,* Vol. II (Washington, D.C.: U.S. Government Printing Office, 1949), pp. 181 ff.

The Declaration of Geneva of the World Medical Association binds the doctor with the words: 'The health of my patient will be my first consideration' and the International Code of Medical Ethics declares that 'Any act or advice which could weaken the physical or mental resistance of a human being may be used only in his interest.'

Because it is essential that the results of laboratory experiments be applied to human beings to further scientific knowledge and to help suffering humanity, the World Medical Association has prepared the following recommendations as a guide to each doctor in clinical research. It must be stressed that the standards as drafted are only a guide to physicians all over the world. Doctors are not relieved from criminal, civil and ethical responsibilities under the laws of their countries.

In the field of clinical research a fundamental distinction must be recognized between clinical research in which the aim is essentially therapeutic for a patient, and the clinical research, the essential object of which is purely scientific and without therapeutic value to the person subjected to research.

I. BASIC PRINCIPLES

1. Clinical research must conform to the moral and scientific principles that justify medical research and should be based on laboratory and animal experiments or other scientifically established facts.
2. Clinical research should be conducted only by scientifically qualified persons and under the supervision of a qualified medical man.
3. Clinical research cannot legitimately be carried out unless the importance of the objectives is in proportion to the inherent risk to the subject.
4. Every clinical research project should be preceded by careful assessment of inherent risks in comparison to foreseeable benefits to the subject.
5. Special caution should be exercised by the doctor in performing clinical research in which the personality of the subject is liable to be altered by drugs or experimental procedure.

II. CLINICAL RESEARCH COMBINED WITH PROFESSIONAL CARE

1. In the treatment of the sick person, the doctor must be free to use a new therapeutic measure, if in his judgment it offers hope of saving life, re-establishing health, or alleviating suffering.

   If at all possible, consistent with patient psychology, the doctor should obtain the patient's freely given consent after the patient has been given a full explanation. In case of legal incapacity, consent should also be procured from the legal guardian; in case of physical incapacity the permission of the legal guardian replaces that of the patient.

2. The doctor can combine clinical research with professional care, the objective being the acquisition of new medical knowledge, only to the extent that clinical research is justified by its therapeutic value for the patient.

III. NON-THERAPEUTIC CLINICAL RESEARCH

1. In the purely scientific application of clinical research carried out on a human being, it is the duty of the doctor to remain the protector of the life and health of that person on whom clinical research is being carried out.

2. The nature, the purpose and the risk of clinical research must be explained to the subject by the doctor.

3a. Clinical research on a human being cannot be undertaken without his free consent after he has been informed; if he is legally incompetent, the consent of the legal guardian should be procured.

3b. The subject of clinical research should be in such a mental, physical and legal state as to be able to exercise fully his power of choice.

3c. Consent should, as a rule, be obtained in writing. However, the responsibility for clinical research always remains with the research worker; it never falls on the subject even after consent is obtained.

4a. The investigator must respect the right of each individual to safeguard his personal integrity, especially if the subject is in a dependent relationship to the investigator.

4b. At any time during the course of clinical research the subject or his guardian should be free to withdraw permission for research to be continued.

The investigator or the investigating team should discontinue the research if in his or their judgment, it may, if continued, be harmful to the individual.

2. *Decisive ethical perspectives*

A medical code does not automatically achieve its goal by the fact that it is well thought out and officially proposed as a set of laws guiding professional behaviour through fear of eventual sanctions. The most fundamental condition for its effectiveness is its capacity to inspire and to find strong convictions and correlative attitudes among the members of the medical profession. In the matter of experimentation, the primary stipulation should be that all investigations be undertaken in absolute responsibility for the individual person, in awareness of the final goal of research and the limits indicated by it. The immediate intention of medical experimentation must always be progress in medical science and practice.

At this point it may help to recall the fundamental perspective of medical ethics, namely, the question, 'what is the meaning of life, health, death, and therefore, the concept of medicine?' True medical progress resides only in that which inscribes itself positively in the whole history of human freedom and liberation. Even the deliverance of mankind from pestilence or epidemics cannot be bought at the price of debasement of the medical profession or indignity to the human person. Health and the liberation of mankind from viral enemies may impose certain restrictions, but we must never lose sight of the greater goal of full development of the person in his capacity to love and to fulfil social responsibilities.

Medical experimentation is, in a way, an expression of the solidarity of mankind. In another way, it can either express full freedom in the manifestation of this solidarity or an undue limitation of freedom for a depersonalizing collectivism. Man matures through openness to the other and to the greater community. Anyone who selflessly and generously chooses to serve the community has attained maturity; he is a whole man. But he who manipulates others by making them instruments for the attainment of his own goals not only violates them as persons, but in the process destroys his own dignity as a person. Regardless of the plausibility of the end, in accumulating scientific data, this attitude portends decay. This is particularly true when a physician, whose profession devotes him to the service of life and the dignity of man, allows himself to choose a course of action abusive of patients and serving only his scientific ambitions.

3. *The patient as experimental subject*

The doctor-patient partnership and the climate of trust and respect so basic for therapy cannot justify the use of a patient as mere experimental subject. The Code of Helsinki emphasizes that the doctor must be free to use a new therapeutic measure if in his judgment it offers hope of saving life, re-establishing health, or alleviating suffering (II, 1), but such an initiative is to be undertaken specifically with a view to serving the patient as a unique person and not as a tool for experimentation. The lesser the chances that traditional and proved methods will be effective, the more easily justifiable will be the truly competent doctor's daring new ways. A decisive criterion therefore is the proportion between hope of success, advantages not so much for the whole of humanity as for the patient and the eventual risk of harmful results for the patient. The physician must guard against using the Code words 'hope' and 'in his judgment' as 'escape words'.[71] He should not even invite his patient to volunteer as subject for medical experiments if the experiments are not truly in the patient's own interests, that is, if they do not actually offer a chance of promoting his health or saving his life.

---

[71] Cf.: Lloyd M. Nyhus, 'Human Experimentation and the Surgeon,' *Surgery*, 64 (October, 1968), 703.

We need therefore to distinguish sharply between experimentation *per se* and the 'therapeutic experiment.' If physicians would systematically record and communicate the results of their therapeutic experiments, they would contribute greatly to the progress of medicine and render more easily dispensable many of the non-therapeutic experiments.

4. *Conditions for non-therapeutic experimentation on human beings*

Most medical codes and civic legislations state unambiguously the basic conditions for outright experimentation on human beings. Laboratory studies, animal experiments and experimental trials of all kinds have to be exhausted before new methods can be applied to human beings. There must furthermore be evidence, or a realistic prospect, of relevance for medical science and practice. Experimentation should be conducted only by highly qualified teams, and the proportion between the risk and hoped-for progress must be sufficiently ascertained. It would be senseless to take considerable risks for unimportant results. The programme should be most carefully planned, after which it should normally be proposed for evaluation by competent non-participants in the projected research. The latter should be allowed to pursue an ongoing evaluation.

In the history of medical progress, self-experimentation by doctors has played an important *rôle*. From a moral point of view, a considerable risk to one's own health and life is more easily justified than the exposure of others to experimental risks. Self-experimentation, however, is not always possible and does not always yield the desired information, especially if a whole series of experiments are required to probe the effectiveness of new techniques. It is considered a valuable criterion not to invite others to cooperate when the investigator himself would not like to be an experimental subject or would not dare invite members of his own family or personal friends to volunteer for the project.

With respect to risk, we have to keep in mind that a great

number of human activities in the technical realm and in the service of others include a sizable risk to health or even to life. Why then, should a well-calculated and well-measured risk through experimentation be excluded? The history of highway construction and bridge spanning has demanded more sacrifices and loss of lives than did any reasonable experimentation in medicine so far. As long as the risk remains within prudent limits, it constitutes a genuine and important service of love in human brotherhood.

Most decisive for the ethical value and moral justification of the risk is the *informed consent* of the volunteers. The Nuremberg Code states that 'the voluntary consent of the human subject is absolutely essential.' This means that the person involved should have legal capacity to give consent, should be so situated as to be able to exercise free choice without the intervention of any element of force, fraud, deceit, duress, or other ulterior form of constraint or coercion. He should have sufficient knowledge and comprehension of the experimental purpose and process to enable him to make an enlightened decision. In other words, before the acceptance of an affirmative decision by the experimental subject, there should be disclosure of: the nature, duration, and purpose of the experiment; the method and means by which it is to be conducted; all inconveniences and hazards reasonably to be expected; and the effects upon his health or person which may possibly come from his participation in the experiment. The duty and responsibility for ascertaining the quality of the consent rests upon each individual who initiates, directs or engages in the experiment. It is a personal duty and responsibility which may not be delegated to another with impunity.

No formulation of a medical code, whatever be its precision, will be effective unless the experimenter is deeply convinced of the dignity of the human person and profoundly respectful of the freedom of consent. There is a vast difference between extorting consent by overwhelming psychological suggestion through cleverly chosen information and gaining consent through completely objective information presented in such a way as to invite the full exercise of judgment and freedom. Those who volunteer as subjects should be encouraged to consult their own physician or spiritual adviser. Neurotics and psychopaths should normally be excluded as experimental subjects since in most cases they are unable to consent freely; besides, they may not prove supportive of the whole experimental process. The investigating team should select candidates chiefly on the basis of their suitability for the particular experiment from a medical viewpoint. It would be desirable that persons outside the research group cooperate not only in the choice of volunteers but also share in the informing process and the continuing moral evaluation of whether or not the experiment, for a certain person, should be carried further or stopped.

Often, there is grave reason to doubt the freedom of consent when the experimental subjects are dependents or students of the experimenting professor. Similarly, much discussion has been reported relative to the cooperation of prisoners as experimental subjects. The prevailing feeling is that there exists no reason for absolute exclusion of prisoners from experimentation if, in healthy self-respect, they truly experience freedom of consent and can judge the relevance of their cooperation with a programme that may yield most significant results for mankind. There must be absolute assurance, however, that the prisoners have the same rights as other persons. They are entitled to receive honest and objective information, and no suggestion or pressure must be brought to bear upon them. The dignity of the human person must be so thoroughly respected that prisoners will never be 'used' as instruments for the attainment of a goal.

The use of mentally retarded persons for non-therapeutic experimentation is extremely problematic since they are unable to give informed consent. They are already in a most pitiable situation and their very condition should dissuade anyone from using them as experimental subjects. Faced with such an inarticulate group, the experimental team would be even more inclined to consider them merely as means and to disregard their dignity as persons. As to relevant experimentation on monsters lacking in human consciousness of any kind and totally incapable of ever attaining it, there can be serious discussions, because experimentation would not infringe on their consciousness and freedom, nor harm them on the personal level.

Ramsey forcefully vetoes any kind of non-therapeutic experimentation with *children*. Most medical codes require informed consent on the part of the parents or legal guardians. On principle, I agree with Ramsey when he challenges the right of parents and tutors to give 'consent on another's behalf, that this other become subject of investigation primarily for the accumulation of scientific knowledge.' [72] In my opinion, he justly insists that besides informed parental or guardian consent, a second condition should also be fulfilled, namely, that the medical investigation bear a definite relation to the treatment of the individual child and promise some advantage to him. Although such a principle poses severe limits on medical experimentation with children, I believe that Ramsey deserves support or at least serious consideration. If he remains inflexible even where there is no 'discernible risk,' [73] I feel that a number of opinions are admissible. Responsible persons need to be wary lest the person of the child be *used* to serve goals other than medical service. No one can better guard the ideal of absolute respect for the human person than the medical profession whose service to humanity is fulfilled in a climate of absolute respect and freedom as expressed in the partnership between doctor and patient.

---

[72] P. Ramsey, *The Patient as Person, op. cit.,* p. 20.
[73] *Ibid.,* p. 39.

BIBLIOGRAPHY

GENERAL

Allwohn, Adolf. *Evangelische Pastoralmedizin.* Stuttgart: Evangelisches, Verlagswerk, 1970.

Babbie, Earl R. *Science and Morality in Medicine: A Survey of Medical Educators.* Berkeley: University of California Press, 1970.

Balint, Michael. *The Doctor, His Patient and Illness.* New York: International Universities Press, 1957.

Belgum, David (ed.). *Religion and Medicine.* Ames, Iowa: Iowa State University Press, 1967.

Biology and Ethics: Proceedings of a Symposium Held at the Royal Geographical Society, London, on September 26-27, 1968. (ed. F.J. Ebling). London-New York: Academic Press, 1969.

Brewer, Lyman A. 'De Humanitate,' *The American Journal of Surgery,* 118, (August, 1969), 133-140.

Browne, T. *Religio Medici,* 1642. London: George Bell and Sons, 1898.

Cadbury, H.J., L. Cleveland et al. *Who Shall Live? Man's Control Over Birth and Death.* A report prepared for the American Friends Service Committee. New York: Hill and Wang, 1970.

Ciba Symposium. *Ethics in Medical Progress.* Boston: Little, Brown and Co., 1966.

Clark-Kennedy, A.E. *Man, Medicine and Morality.* London: Faber and Faber, 1969.

Clayton, Ernest and H.A. McKay. *Medicine, Morals and Man.* New York: International Publications Service, 1969.

Curran, Charles E. *Contemporary Problems in Moral Theology.* Notre Dame: Fides Publishers, 1970.

Cutler, D.R. (ed.). *Updating Life and Death: Essays in Ethics and Medicine.* Boston: Beacon Press, 1969.

Daly, Cahal B. *Morals, Law and Life.* Chicago: Scepter Publisher, 1966.

DeGroot, L.J. *Medical Care: Social and Organizational Aspects.* Springfield, Ill.: C.C. Thomas Publishers, 1966.

Deutsch, Felix (ed.). *Training in Psychosomatic Medicine.* New York: Hafner Publishers, 1964.

DeWolf, L. Harold. *Responsible Freedom.* New York: Harper & Row, 1971.

Dubos, René. *Man Adapting.* New Haven and London: Yale University Press, 1965.

Edmunds, V. *The Changing Face of Medical Ethics.* Conference of European Physicians. Amsterdam, 1965.

Edmunds, V. and C.G. Scorer (eds.). *Ethical Responsibility in Medicine: A Christian Approach.* Edinburgh-London: E. & S. Livingston, Ltd., 1967.

Fletcher, Joseph. *Morals and Medicine.* Boston: Beacon Press, 1960.

219

Galdston, Iago (ed.) *Institute of Social and Historical Medicine.* New York: International Universities Press.
  I: *On the Utility of Medical History* (1958)
 II: *The Impact of Antibiotics on Medicine and Society* (1969)
III: *Human Nutrition, Historic and Scientific* (1961)
 IV: *Man's Image in Medicine and Anthropoloy* (1963).
Galdston, Iago. *Medicine in Transition.* Chicago: University of Chicago Press, 1965.
Gustafson, James M. 'Basic ethical issues in the bio-medical fields,' *Soundings,* 53 (1970), 151-180.
Häring, Bernard. *Hope is the Remedy.* Slough: St Paul Publications, 1971.
Häring, Bernard. *Morality is for Persons.* New York: Farrar-Straus-Giroux, 1971.
Healy, Edwin F. *Medical Ethics.* Loyola University Press, 1956.
Hyde, Margaret O. *Medicine in Action: Today and Tomorrow.* New York: McGraw-Hill, 1964.
Jakobovitz, Immanuel. *Jewish Medical Ethics.* New York: Bloch Publishing Co., 1959.
Johnson, Paul. *Psychologie der pastoralen Beratung.* Wien: Herder, 1969.
Jores, Arthur. *Die Medizin in der Krise unserer Zeit.* Stuttgart: Hans Huber, 1966.
Jores, Arthur. *Um eine Medizin von Morgen.* Bern: Verlag Hans Huber, 1969.
Jores, Arthur. *Wrote für Kranke.* Bern: Verlag Hans Huber, 1969.
Kaufman, M. Ralph and Marcel Heiman. *Evolution of Psychosomatic Concepts.* New York: International Universities Press, 1964.
Kelly, Gerald. *Medico-Moral Problems.* St Louis: Catholic Hospital Association, 1958.
Kenny, John P. *Principles of Medical Ethics* (2nd ed.) Westminster, Md.: Newman Press, 1962.
King, Maurice H. (ed.), *Medical Care in Developing Countries.* New York: Oxford University Press, 1966.
Labby, D.H. (ed.). *Life or Death: Ethics and Options.* Portland, Ore.: Reed College; Seattle and London: University of Washington Press, 1968.
Lasagna, Louis. *Life, Death and the Doctor.* New York: Alfred Knopf, 1968.
Macquarrie, John. *Three Issues in Ethics.* New York: Harper and Row, 1970.
Marshall, J. *The Ethics of Medical Practice.* London: Darton-Longman-Todd, 1960.
McFadden C., *Medical Ethics* (6th ed.). Philadelphia: Davis, 1967.
McKeown, Thomas and C.R. Lowe. *Introduction to Social Medicine.* Philadelphia: Blackwell Davis Co., 1966.
Niedermeyer, Albert. *Compendium of Pastoral Medicine.* (trans. Fulgence Buonanno). New York: Joseph F. Wagner, 1961.
O'Donnell, T. *Morals in Medicine* (2nd ed.). Westminster, Md.: Newman Press, 1960.

Ramsey, Paul. *The Patient as Person.* New Haven: Yale University Press, 1970.

Reagan, Charles E. *Ethics for Scientific Researchers.* (2nd ed.) Springfield, Ill.: Charles C. Thomas, 1971.

Regau, Th. *Medizin auf Abwegen. Der Einbruch der Technik in die Heilkunst.* München, 1960.

Rhoads, Paul S. 'Medical ethics and morals in a new age,' *Journal of the American Medical Association,* 205 (August, 1968), 517-522.

Smith, Harmon L. *Ethics and the New Medicine.* Nashville: Abingdon Press, 1970.

Snoeck, Andre. *Mental Hygiene and Christian Principles.* Cork: Mercier Press, 1962.

Sperry, Willard L. *The Ethical Basis of Medical Practice.* New York: Harper and Bros., Paul B. Hoeber, 1956.

Strauss, Anselm L. (ed.) *Where Medicine Fails.* Trans-action Book Service. No. 4. Chicago: Aldine Publishing Co., 1970.

Torrey, E.F. (ed.) *Ethical Issues in Medicine. The Role of the Physician in Today's Society.* Boston: Little, Brown and Co., 1968.

Tournier, Paul. *Guilt and Grace.* New York: Harper and Row, 1962.

Tournier, Paul. *Krankheit und Lebensprobleme.* Basel: 1965.

Viets, Henry R. *Humanism and the Student of Medicine.* Hanover, N.H.: Dartmouth Publications, 1960.

Webber, Irving L. (ed.). *Medical Care under Social Security. Potentials and Problems.* Gainesville: University of Florida Press, 1966.

Zinberg, Norman E. (ed.). *Psychiatry and Medical Practice in a General Hospital.* New York: International Universities Press, 1964.

CHAPTER 1

Aschner, B. *The Art of the Healer.* New York: Dial Press, 1942.

Barbour, Ian G. (ed.). *Science and Religion: New Perspectives on the Dialogue.* New York: Harper & Row, 1968.

Buck, Albert H. *The Growth of Medicine from the Earliest Times to About 1800.* New Haven. Yale University Press, 1971.

Castiglioni, A. *A History of Medicine.* New York: Knopf, 1947.

Coggeshall, L. *Progress and Paradox on the Medical Scene.* Chicago: University of Chicago Press, 1966.

Galdston, Iago. *Historic Derivations of Modern Psychiatry.* New York: McGraw-Hill, 1967.

Garrison, Fielding H. *An Introduction to the History of Medicine.* Philadelphia: W.B. Saunders, 1929.

Identity and Dignity of Man: A Scientific, Theological, and Humanistic Dialogue on Issues Emerging from Behavioral, Surgical, and Genetic Interventions. (Symposia of the American Association for the Advancement of Science, Boston, December, 1969). Cambridge, Mass.: Schenckman Publishing Co., 1970.

King, L. *The Medical World of the 18th Century.* Chicago: University of Chicago Press, 1958.

Ramsey, Paul. 'The ethics of a cottage industry in an age of community and research medicine,' *New England Journal of Medicine*, 284 (April, 1971), 700-706.

Rivers, W.H.R. *Medicine, Magic and Religion*. New York: Harcourt, 1924.

Sigerist, H.E. *History of Medicine*. 2 vols. New York. Oxford University Press. I. Primitive and Archaic Medicine (1951) II. Early Greek, Hindu and Persian Medicine (1961).

Siirala, M. *Medicine in Metamorphosis: Speech, Presence and Integration*. Tavistock. Barnes and Noble, 1969.

Toffler, Alvin. *Future Shock*. Los Angeles: Western Psychological Services, 1971.

Turner, E.S. *Call the Doctor, a Social History of Medical Men*. New York: St Martin's Press, 1959.

White, D. (ed.). *Dialogue in Medicine and Theology*. Nashville, N.Y.: Abingdon Press, 1967.

CHAPTER 2

Brown, T. 'Essay on Christian morals,' *Religio Medici and Other Writings*. New York: Everyman's Library, Vol. 92 (E.P. Dutton & Co.), 1951.

Francis, Henry S. 'Traditional Representation of Medicine and Healing in the Christian Hierarchy,' *Bulletin of the Medical Library Association*, 32 (July, 1944), 332-334.

The Human Body. Papal teachings; selected and arranged by the Benedictine Monks of Solesmes. Boston: St Paul Editions, 1960.

Long, Edward L., Jr. and Robert T. Handy. *Theology and Church in Times of Change*. Philadelphia: Westminster Press, 1970.

CHAPTER 3

Adams, E. Maynard. *Ethical Naturalism and the Modern World-View*. Chapel Hill: University of No. Carolina Press, 1960.

Curran, Charles E. (ed.) *Absolutes in Moral Theology*. Washington, D.C. and Cleveland: Corpus Books, 1968.

Häring, Bernard. *Christian Existentialist*, New York: New York University Press, 1968.

Häring, Bernard. *The Law of Christ*. 3 vols. Westminster, Md.: Newman Press, 1961-1966.

Higgins, T.J. *Ethical Theories in Conflict*. Milwaukee: Bruce Publishing, 1967.

Hudson, W.D. *Ethical Intuitionism*. New York: St Martin's Press, 1967.

Hudson, W.D. *Modern Moral Philosophy*. Garden City, N.Y.: Doubleday, 1970.

Leake, Chauncey D. 'Theories of ethics and medical practice,' *Journal of the American Medical Association*, 208 (May, 1969), 842-847.

Rader, M. *Ethics and the Human Community.* New York: Holt, Rinehart and Winston, 1964.

Roubiczek, Paul. *Ethical Values in an Age of Science.* New York: Cambridge University Press, 1969.

Shirk, E. *Ethical Dimension: An Approach to the Philosophy of Values and Valuing.* New York: Appleton, 1965.

Smith, Harmon L. *The Christian and His Decisions.* Nashville, N.Y.: Abingdon, 1969.

CHAPTER 4

Alexander, Franz et al. *Psychosomatic Specificity.* Chicago: University of Chicago Press, 1968.

American Medical Association. *Principles of Medical Ethics.* Boston: Massachusetts Medical Society, 1962.

Barton, R.T. 'Sources of medical morals,' *Journal of the American Medical Association,* 193 (July, 1965), 133-138.

Chavez, I. 'Professional ethics in our time,' *Journal of the American Medical Association,* 190 (1964), 226-231.

Eastwood, R.T. et al. *Cardiac Replacement: Medical, Ethical, Psychological and Economic Implications.* (Report by the Ad Hoc Task Force on Cardiac Replacement, National Heart Institute, National Institutes of Health, Public Health Service, U.S. Department of Health, Education and Welfare). Washington, D.C.: Superintendent of Documents, U.S. Government Printing Office, 1969.

Edel, A. *Ethical Judgment: The Use of Science in Ethics.* New York: Free Press, 1955.

Edmunds, V. and C.G. Scorer (eds). *Ethical Responsibility in Medicine: A Christian Approach.* Baltimore: Williams and Williams Co., 1967.

Galdston, Iago. *The Meaning of Social Medicine.* Cambridge, Mass.: Harvard University Press, 1954.

Guttentag, O. 'A course entitled "The Medical Attitude",' *Journal of Medical Education,* 35 (October, 1960), 903-907.

Irish, D.P. and D.W. McMurry, 'Professional oaths and American Medical Colleges,' *Journal of Chronic Diseases,* 18 (March, 1965), 275-289.

Krevans, Julius R. and Peter G. Condliffe (eds). *Reform of Medical Education: The Effect of Student Unrest.* Washington, D.C.: National Academy of Sciences, 1970.

Lyons, Catherine. *Organ Transplants: The Moral Issues.* Philadelphia: Westminster Press, 1970.

MacKinney, Loren M. 'Medical ethics and etiquette in the early middle ages,' *Bulletin of the History of Medicine,* 26 (1952), 1-31.

Massachusetts Medical Society. *Code of Ethics.* Boston: Massachusetts Medical Society, 1962.

National Urban League. *Health Care and the Negro Population.* New York: National Urban League, 1965 (pamphlet).

Norwood, W.F. 'Foundations of professional conduct,' *Medical Arts and Sciences,* 17 (1963), 77-85.

P

One Life — One Physician: An Inquiry into the Medical Profession's Performance in Self-Regulation. (A report to the Centre for Study of Responsive Law by L.T. Keelty et al. and Robert S. McCleery, Project Director). Washington, D.C.: 1970.

Savatier, R. *La responsabilité médicale.* Paris: Lethielleux, 1948.

Silver, G.A. *Family Medical Care.* Cambridge, Mass.: Harvard University Press, 1963.

Silver, G.A. 'New types of personnel and changing roles of health professionals,' *Bulletin of the New York Academy of Medicine,* 42 (December, 1966), 1217-1225.

Smith, Harmon L. *Ethics and the New Medicine.* Nashville, N.Y.: Abingdon, 1970.

Tiberghien, P. *Médecine et morals, Les devoirs généraux du médecin.* Paris-Tournai-Rome: Desclée, 1952.

Wise, Harold B. 'Medicine and poverty,' *Ethical Issues in Medicine* (ed. E.F. Torrey). Boston: Little, Brown and Co., 1968. 347-370.

'Zum deontologischen Gehalt ärtzlicher Standesordnungen,' *Arzt und Christ,* 17 (1971), 1-41.

CHAPTER 5

Barlow, P. and C.G. Vosa. 'The Y chromosome in human spermatozoa,' *Nature* (London), 226 (1970), 961-962.

Baruk, H. *La désorganisation de la personnalité.* Paris, 1952.

Caruso, I.A. *Bios, Psyche, Person.* Freiburg-München, 1957.

Curran, Charles E. 'Moral theology and genetics,' *Cross Currents,* XX (Winter, 1970), 64-82.

Delgado, José M.R. 'Evaluation of electrical control of the brain,' Part IV in *Physical Control of the Mind.* New York: Harper & Row, 1969, 180-230.

Diasio, R.E. and R.H. Glass. 'The Y chromosome in sperm of an XYY male,' *Lancet,* 2 (1970), 1318-1319.

Dobzhansky, Theodosius. *Heredity and the Nature of Man.* New York: Harcourt, Brace & World, 1964.

Dubos, R.J. 'The philosophy of medicine in 1985,' *What's New,* 220 (1961), 4-5.

Genetic Counselling: Third Report of the WHO Expert Committee on Human Genetics. (WHO Technical Reports Series, § 416). Geneva: World Health Organization, 1969.

Heschel, Abraham J. 'The patient as a person,' in *Insecurity of Freedom. Essays on Human Existence.* New York: Farrar, Straus & Giroux, 1966.

Heschel, Abraham J. *Who is Man?* Stanford: Stanford University Press, 1965.

Hulten, M. and P.L. Pearson. 'Fluorescent evidence for spermatocytes with two Y chromosomes in an XYY male,' *Annals of Human Genetics* 34 (1971), 273-276.

Lawrence, L. *Were We Controlled?* New Hyde Park: University Books, 1967.
'Medicine in the year 2000.' *Report of Proceedings: Sixth Annual Conference on Graduate Medical Education.* Philadelphia: University of Penn. School of Medicine, 1964.
Moore, G.E. 'Biological ethics; the fantastic future,' *California Medicine,* 109 (December, 1968), 494-498.
Mouroux, J. *The Meaning of Man* (trans. A.H.G. Downes). New York: Doubleday — Image Books, 1961.
Parker, W. Carey and Alexander G. Bearn. 'Application of genetic regulatory mechanisms to human genetics,' *American Journal of Medicine,* 34 (May, 1963), 680-691.
Ramsey, Paul. *Fabricated Man: The Ethics of Genetic Control.* New Haven: Yale University Press, 1970.
Rohrer, Wolf. *Ist der Mensch konstruierbar?* Munich: Verlag Ars Sacra, 1966.
Rorvik, David M. and Landrum B. Shettles. *Your Baby's Sex: Now You Can Choose.* New York: Dodd, Mead and Co., 1970.
Rotter, Hans. 'Die Manipulation das Menschen,' *Arzt und Christ,* 16 (1970), 21-29.
Sigerist, H.E. *Medicine and Human Welfare.* College Park, Md.: McGrath-Publishing Co., 1941.
Summer, A.T., J.A. Robinson and H.J. Evans. 'Distinguishing between X, Y, and YY-bearing human spermatozoa by Fluorescence and DNA content,' *Nature: New Biology,* 229 (1971), 231-233.
Tillich, Paul. *The Courage To Be.* New Haven: Yale University Press, 1952.
Tillich, Paul. *Love, Power and Justice: Ontological Analyses and Ethical Applications.* New York: Oxford University Press, 1960.
Wolstenholme, G. (ed.) *Man and His Future.* Boston: Little, Brown and Co., 1963.

CHAPTER 6

Abortion: An Ethical Discussion. The Church and Assembly Board for Social Responsibility. London: Church (of England) Information Office, 1965.
Advisory Board on Sex, Marriage and the Family, British Council of Churches. *The Abortion Act, 1967-69. A Factual Review.* London: Witney Press, 1970.
Augenstein, Leroy. *Come, Let Us Play God.* New York: Harper and Row, 1969.
Barrett, Donald N. (ed.). *The Problem of Population.* Vol. I: *Moral and Theological Considerations.* Notre Dame, Ind.: University of Notre Dame Press, 1964.
Berg, J.M. (ed.). *Genetic Counselling in Relation to Mental Retardation.* New York. Pergamon Press, 1971.
Behrman, S.J. 'Artificial insemination,' *International Journal of Fertility,* 6 (1961), 291-297.

Berrill, N.J. *The Person in the Womb.* New York: Dodd, Mead and Co., 1968.

Burke, C. 'Abortion: law ethics and the value of life,' *Manchester Medical Gazette,* 49 (July, 1970), 4-9.

Burke, W.T. 'Abortion and the psychiatrist,' *The Homiletic and Pastoral Review,* LXXI (December, 1970), 199-207.

Callahan, Daniel. *Abortion: Law, Choice and Morality.* New York: Macmillan, 1970.

Callahan, Daniel (ed.) *The Catholic Case for Contraception.* New York: Macmillan Company, 1969.

Contemporary Themes 'The abortion act (1967),' *British Medical Journal,* (May 30, 1970), 529-535.

Cooke, R.E., A.E. Hellegers et al. (eds.) *The Terrible Choice: The Abortion Dilemma.* New York: Bantam Books, 1968.

Curran, Charles E. (ed.) *Contraception: Authority and Dissent.* New York: Herder and Herder, 1964.

Curran, Charles E. 'Moral theology and genetics,' *Cross Currents,* 20 (1970), 64-82.

Curran, Charles E. 'Theology and genetics: a multi-faceted dialogue,' *Journal of Ecumenical Studies,* 7 (1970), 61-89.

Darlington, C.D. *Genetics and Man.* New York: Schoken Books, 1969.

De Chardin, Teilhard. 'The birth of thought,' in *The Phenomenon of Man.* New York: Harper and Row, 1965. Pp. 163-190.

Dobzhansky, Theodosius. *The Biology of Ultimate Concern.* New York: New American Library, 1967.

Dobzhansky, Theodosius. 'Evolution: implications for religion,' *Christian Century,* 84 (July 19, 1967), 936-941.

Donceel, J.F. 'Immediate animation and delayed hominization,' *Theological Studies,* 31 (1970), 76-105.

Dupre, Louis K. *Contraception and Catholics: A New Appraisal.* Baltimore: Helicon Press, 1964.

Eastman, N.J. and L.M. Hellman. *Obstetrics.* (13th ed.) New York: Appleton-Century-Crofts 1966.

Edwards, R.G. and Ruth E. Fowler. 'Human embryos in the laboratory,' *Scientific American,* 223 (1970), 45-54.

Feldman, David M. *Birth Control in Jewish Law.* New York: New York University Press, 1968.

Finegold, Wilfred J. 'Artificial insemination,' in *Ethical Issues in Medicine* (ed. E.F. Torrey), Boston. Little, Brown and Co., 1968. 53-73.

Finegold, Wilfred J. *Artificial Insemination.* Springfield, Ill.: Charles C. Thomas, 1964.

Flood, Peter. 'Abortion,' in *New Problems in Medical Ethics.* IV. Cork: Ireland. Mercier Press, 1963. 9-60.

Francoeur, T. *Utopian Motherhood: New Trends in Human Reproduction.* New York: Doubleday, 1970.

Glass, Bentley. 'Human Heredity and Ethical Problems,' First Annual Address to the Society for Health and Human Values, (October 29, 1970), Los Angeles.

Granfield, David. *The Abortion Decision*. Garden City, N.Y.: Doubleday, 1969.

Grisez, Germain G. *Abortion: The Myths, the Realities and the Arguments*. New York: Corpus Publishing, 1970.

Gustafson, James M. 'Context versus principles. A displaced debate in Christian ethics,' *The Harvard Theological Review*, 58 (1965), 171-202.

Gustafson, James M. 'A Protestant ethical approach,' in *The Morality of Abortion* (ed. J.T. Noonan, Jr.). Cambridge, Mass.: Harvard University Press, 1970. 101-122.

Guttmacher, A.F. 'Contraception,' *Ethical Issues in Medicine* (ed. E.F. Torrey). Boston: Little, Brown and Co., 1968. 25-51.

Guttmacher, A.F., 'Intra-uterine contraceptive devices,' *Journal of Reproduction and Fertility*, 10 (August, 1965), 115-128.

Guttmacher, A.F. W. Best and F. Jaffe. *Planning Your Family*. New York: Macmillan, 1965.

Handler, Philip (ed.) *Biology and the Future of Man*. New York: Oxford University Press, 1970.

Hall, Robert E. (ed.) *Abortion in a Changing World*. 2 vols. New York: Columbia University Press, 1970.

Hardin, Garrett (ed.). *Population, Evolution and Birth Control: A Collage of Controversial Readings*. (2nd ed.) San Francisco: W.H. Freeman & Co., 1969.

Häring, Bernard. *Love is the Answer*. Danville, N.J.: Dimension Books, 1970.

Häring, Bernard. 'A theological evaluation,' in *The Morality of Abortion* (ed. J.T. Noonan, Jr.). Cambridge, Mass.: Harvard University Press, 1970. 123-145.

Harris, Peter et al. *On Human Life*. London: Burns and Oates, 1968.

Heath, D.S. 'Psychiatry and Abortion,' *Canadian Psychiatric Association Journal*, 16 (1971) 55-63.

Hellegers, A.E. 'Fetal development,' *Theological Studies*, 31 (1970), 3-9.

Himes, N.E. *Medical History of Contraception*. New York: Gamut Press, 1963.

Hoyt, Robert G. (ed.). *The Birth Control Debate*. Kansas City: National Catholic Reporter Publishing Co., 1968.

Huisingh, Donald. 'Should man control his genetic future?' *Zygon*, 4 (1969), 188-199.

Kindregan, Charles P. *Abortion, the Law and Defective Children: A Legal-Medical Study*. New York: Corpus Publishing, 1969.

Knutson, Andie L. 'When does a human life begin? Viewpoints of public health professionals,' *American Journal of Public Health*, 57 (December, 1967), 2163-2177.

Lader, Lawrence. *Abortion*. New York: Beacon Press, 1966.

Lederberg, Joshua. 'Experimental genetics and human evolution,' *Bulletin of Atomic Sciences*, 22 (1966), 4-11.

Lederberg, Joshua. 'Genetic engineering and the amelioration of genetic defect,' *Biosciences*, 20 (1970), 1307-1310.

Maris, Ronald W. *Social Forces in Urban Suicide.* Homewood, Ill.: Dorsey Press, 1969.

Milhaven, J.G. 'The abortion debate: an epistemological interpretation,' *Theological Studies,* 31 (1970), 106-124.

Noonan, John T. Jr. 'An almost absolute value in history,' in *The Morality of Abortion* (ed. J.T. Noonan, Jr.). Cambridge, Mass.: Harvard University Press, 1970. 1-59.

Noonan, John T. Jr. *Contraception: A History of Its Treatment by Catholic Theologians and Canonists.* Toronto and New York: New American Library, 1967.

Noonan, John T. Jr., (ed.) *The Morality of Abortion.* Cambridge, Mass.: Harvard University Press, 1970.

O'Brien, John A. et al. *Family Planning in an Exploding Population.* New York: Hawthorne Books, 1968.

Overhage, P. and K. Rahner. *Das Problem der Homonisation* (Questiones disputatae 12/13). Freiburg, 1961.

Paterson, David, (ed.) *Genetic Engineering.* London: British Broadcasting Corporation, 1969.

Paul VI, Pope. *Humanae Vitae: On the Regulation of Birth.* New York: Paulist Press, 1968.

Quinn, Francis K. (ed.) *Population Ethics.* Washington, D.C.: Corpus Books, 1968.

Riga, Peter J. 'Modern science and the ethical dimension,' *Catholic World,* 209 (1969), 213-217.

Robinson, Daniel N., (ed.). *Heredity and Achievement: A Book of Readings.* New York: Oxford University Press, 1970.

Rock, John. *The Time Has Come: A Catholic Doctor's Proposals to End the Battle over Birth Control.* New York: Alfred A. Knopf, 1963.

Rorvik, David M. *Brave New Baby: Promise and Peril of the Biological Revolution.* Garden City, N.Y.: Doubleday and Co., 1971.

Rorvik, David M. 'Taking life in our hands: the test-tube baby is coming,' *Look,* (May 18, 1971), 83-88.

Rosen, Harold (ed.) *Abortion in America.* Boston: Beacon Press, 1967.

Rosenfeld, Albert. *The Second Genesis: The Coming Control of Life.* Englewood Cliffs, N.J.: Prentice-Hall, 1969.

Rosenthal, David. *Genetic Theory and Abnormal Behavior.* New York: McGraw-Hill Book Co., 1970.

Roslansky, John D., (ed.) *Genetics and the Future of Man: A Discussion at the Nobel Conference Organized by Gustavus Adolphus College, St Peter, Minnesota, 1965.* Amsterdam: North Holland Publishing Co., 1966.

Rostand, Jean. *Can Man Be Modified?* (trans. J. Griffin). New York: Basic Books, 1959.

St John-Stevas, Norman. *The Right to Life.* New York: Holt, Rinehart and Winston, 1964.

Schwartz, R.A., 'Psychiatry and the abortion laws: an overview,' *Comprehensive Psychiatry,* 9 (1968), 99-117.

Shannon, William H. *The Lively Debate: Response to Humanae Vitae.* New York: Sheed and Ward, 1970.

Shinn, Roger L., 'Genetic decisions: a case study in ethical method,' *Soundings,* 52 (1969), 299-310.

Shuster, George N. (ed.). *The Problem of Population.* Vol. II. *Practical Catholic Application.* Notre Dame, Ind.: University of Notre Dame Press, 1964.

Simon, N.M. et al. 'Psychological factors related to spontaneous and therapeutic abortion,' *American Journal of Obstetrics and Gynecology,* 104 (July, 1969), 799-808.

Smith, David T., (ed.). *Abortion and the Law.* Cleveland: Press of Case-Western Reserve University, 1967.

Sonnenborn, T.M. (ed.). *The Control of Human Heredity and Evolution.* New York: Macmillan, 1965.

Taylor, Gordon R. *The Biological Time Bomb.* Signet Books. New York: New American Library, 1968.

Tietze, C. 'Effectiveness and acceptability of intra-uterine contraceptive devices,' *American Journal of Public Health,* 55 (1965), 1874 ff.

Tietze, C. 'Some facts about legal abortion,' *Human Fertility and Population Problems* (ed. R.O. Greep). Cambridge, Mass.: Schenkman Publishers, 1963.

Tyler, E.T. *Sterility.* New York: McGraw-Hill, 1961.

Vauj, K. (ed.). *Who Shall Live? Medicine-Technology-Ethics.* Philadelphia: Fortress Press, 1970.

Viola, Michael V. 'Abortion: a Catholic View,' *Ethical Issues in Medicine* (ed. E.F. Torrey). Boston: Little, Brown and Co., 1968. 87-104.

Warshofsky, Fred. *The Control of Life in the 21st Century.* New York: Viking Press, 1967.

Wood, H.C. *Sex Without Babies.* Philadelphia: Whitmore Publishing Co., 1967.

Wood, H.C. 'Sterilization,' in *Ethical Issues in Medicine* (ed. E.F. Torrey). Boston: Little Brown and Co., 1968. 105-137.

Zuspan, Frederick P. (ed.) 'Pregnancy termination: the impact of new laws,' *Journal of Reproductive Medicine,* 6 (1971), 274-301.

CHAPTER 7

Aring, Charles D. 'Intimations of morality: an appreciation of death and dying,' *Annals of Internal Medicine,* 69 (July, 1968), 137-152.

Baltzell, William H. 'The dying patient. When the focus must be changed,' *Archives of Internal Medicine,* 127 (January, 1971), 106-109.

Beecher, Henry K. et al. 'A definition of irreversible coma,' *Journal of the American Medical Association,* 205 (August, 1968), 85-88.

Beecher, Henry K. 'Definitions of "life" and "death" for medical science and practice,' *Annals of the New York Academy of Sciences,* 169 (January, 1970), 471-474.

Beecher, Henry K. 'Ethical problems created by the hopelessly unconscious patient,' *New England Journal of Medicine,* 278 (1968), 1425-1430.

Berman, Merrill I. 'The Todeserwartung syndrome,' *Geriatrics,* 21 (May, 1966), 187-192.

Biörck, Gunnar. 'Thoughts on life and death,' *Perspectives in Biology and Medicine,* 2 (Summer, 1968), 527-543.

Blauner, Robert. 'Death and the social structure,' *Psychiatry,* 29 (November, 1966), 378-394.

Boros, Ladislaus. *The Mystery of Death.* New York: Herder and Herder, 1965.

Brim, Orville G. et al. *The Dying Patient.* New York: Russell Sage Foundation, 1970.

Carroll, C. 'The ethics of heart transplantation,' *Journal of the National Medical Association,* 62 (January, 1970), 14-20.

Childress, James. 'Who shall live when not all can live?' *Soundings,* 53 (1970), 339-362.

Choron, Jacques. *Death and Western Thought.* New York: Collier, 1963.

Choron, Jacques. *Modern Man and Mortality.* New York: Macmillan, 1964.

Cleland, J.T. (ed.). 'The right to live and the right to die,' *Medical Times,* 95 (1967), 1171-1196.

Collins, Vincent J. 'Limits of medical responsibility in prolonging life,' *Journal of the American Medical Association,* 206 (October, 1968), 389-392.

Downing, A.B., (ed.). *Euthanasia and the Right to Death: The Case for Voluntary Euthanasia.* London: Peter Owen, 1969.

Drinan, Robert F. 'Should there be a legal right to die?' *American Ecclesiastical Review,* 159 (1968), 277-286.

Dubost, Charles. 'Scientific and ethical problems in organ transplantation,' *Annals of Thoracic Surgery,* 8 (August, 1969), 95-103.

Dukeminier, Jesse, Jr. and D. Sanders. 'Organ transplantation. A proposal for routine salvaging of cadaver organs,' *New England Journal of Medicine,* 279 (August, 1968), 413-419.

Easson, William M. *The Dying Child: The Management of the Child or Adolescent Who Is Dying.* Springfield, Ill.: Charles C. Thomas, 1970.

Eaton, Joseph W. 'The art of aging and dying,' *The Gerontologist,* 4 (June, 1964), 94-100.

Elkinton, J.R. 'When do we let the patient die?' *Annals of Internal Medicine,* 68 (1968), 695-700.

Feder, Samuel L. 'Attitudes of patients with advanced malignancy,' *Symposium of the Group for the Advancement of Psychiatry,* 5 (October, 1965), 614-622.

Feifel, Herman, (ed.). *The Meaning of Death.* New York: McGraw-Hill, 1959.

Feifel, Herman et al. 'Physicians consider death,' *Proceedings of the 75th Annual Convention of the American Psychological Association,* 2 (1967), 201-202.

Fishgold, H. 'Electroencephalographe et signes de la mort,' *Cahiers Laennec* (September, 1970), 48-53.

Friedman, S.B. et al. 'Behavioral observations on parents anticipating the death of a child,' *Pediatrics*, 32 (October, 1963), 610-625.

Fulton, Robert (ed.). *Death and Identity*. New York: John Wiley & Sons, 1965.

Gatch, Milton. *Death: Meaning and Mortality in Christian Thought and Contemporary Culture*. New York: Seabury Press, 1969.

Glaser, Barney G. and A.L. Strauss. *Awareness of Dying*. Chicago: Aldine Press, 1965.

Glaser, Barney G. 'Disclosure of terminal illness,' *Journal of Health and Human Behavior*, 7 (Summer, 1966), 32-91.

Glaser, Barney G. *Time for Dying*. Chicago: Aldine Press, 1968.

Godin, André et al. *Mort et présence*. Bruxelles: Lumen Vitae, 1971.

Gorer, Geoffrey. *Death, Grief and Mourning*. Garden City, N. Y.: Doubleday and Co., 1965.

Grollman, Earl A. *Explaining Death to Children*. Boston: Beacon Press, 1967.

Hinton, John M. *Dying*. Baltimore, Md.: Penguin Books, 1967.

Hinton, John M. 'Facing death,' *Journal of Psychosomatic Research*, 10 (July, 1966), 22-28.

Kalish, Richard A. 'The practising physician and death research,' *Medical Times*, 97 (January, 1969), 211-220.

Kastenbaum, Robert and Ruth B. Aisenberg. *The Psychology of Death*. New York: Springer Publishing Co., 1971.

Kübler-Ross, Elizabeth. *On Death and Dying*. New York: Macmillan Co., 1969.

Kutscher, Austin H. (ed.). *Death and Bereavement*. Springfield, Ill.: Charles C. Thomas, 1969.

Laforet, Eugene G. 'The hopeless case,' *Linacre Quarterly*, 29 (1962), 126-143.

Laforet, Eugene G. 'The hopeless case,' *Archives of Internal Medicine*, 112 (1963), 314-326.

Letourneau, Charles U. 'Dying with dignity,' *Hospital Management* (June, 1970), 27, 30.

Lewis, C.S. *The Problem of Pain*. New York: Macmillan, 1962.

McNaspy, C.J. 'Murder for mercy's sake: on killing thalidomide babies,' *America*, 107 (December 15, 1962), 1242-1244.

Meyer, Bernard C. 'Truth and the physician,' *Bulletin of the New York Academy of Medicine*, 45 (January, 1969), 59-71.

Meyer, Bernard C. 'Truth and the physician,' in *Ethical Issues in Medicine* (ed. E.F. Torrey). Boston: Little, Brown and Co., 1968. 159-177.

Mills, Liston (ed.). *Perspectives on Death*. Nashville: Abingdon Press, 1969.

Pearson, Leonard (ed.). *Death and Dying: Current Issues in the Treatment of the Dying Person*. Cleveland: Case Western Reserve Press, 1969.

Perper, J.A. 'Ethical, religious and legal considerations to the transplantation of human organs,' *Journal of Forensic Sciences*, 15 (January, 1970), 1-13.

Pompey, H. 'Gehirntod und totaler Tod,' *Münchener Medizinische Wochenschrift,* 13 (1969), 736-741.

Rahner, Karl. 'Gedanken über das Sterben,' *Arzt und Christ,* 15 (1969), 24-32.

Rahner, Karl. *On the Theology of Death.* New York: Herder and Herder, 1961.

Rapaport, Felix T. and Jean Dausset (eds). *Human Transplantation.* New York: Grune and Stratton, 1968.

Reich, Warren. *Medico-Moral Problems and the Principle of Totality: A Catholic Viewpoint.* Washington, D.C.: Veterans Administration Hospitals, 1967.

Rhoads, Paul S. 'Moral considerations in prolongation of life,' *Journal of the So. Carolina Medical Association* (October, 1968), 422-428.

Ruff, Wilfried. *Organwerpflanzungen. Ethische Probleme aus katholische Sicht.* München: Wilhelm Goldmann Verlag, 1971.

Schoenberg, B. et al. (eds). *Loss and Grief: Psychological Management in Medical Practice.* New York: Columbia University Press, 1970.

Scott, Nathan A., Jr. (ed.) *The Modern Vision of Death.* Richmond, Va.: John Knox Press, 1967.

Sullivan, J.V. *The Morality of Mercy Killing.* Westminster, Md.: Newman Press, 1950.

Vaisrub, S. 'The Fade-out,' *Archives of Internal Medicine,* 121 (June, 1968), 511-517.

Vernon, Glenn M. *Sociology of Death: An Analysis of Death-Related Behavior.* New York: Ronald Press Co., 1970.

Verwaerdt, Adriaam. *Communication with the Fatally Ill.* Springfield, Ill.: Charles C. Thomas, 1966.

Williams, Robert H. 'Our role in the generation, modification and termination of life,' *Archives of Internal Medicine,* 124 (August, 1969), 215-237.

Winter, Arthur (ed.). *The Moment of Death.* Springfield, Ill.: Charles C. Thomas, 1969.

Wolff, Kurt. 'Helping elderly patients face the fear of death,' *Hospital and Community Psychiatry,* 18 (May, 1967), 142-144.

Wolstenholme, G.E.W. and Maeve O'Connor (eds.) *Ethics in Medical Progress: With Special Reference to Transplantation.* Ciba Foundation Symposium. Boston: Little, Brown and Co., 1966.

Zinker, Joseph C. and S.L. Fink. 'The possibility for psychological growth in a dying person,' *Journal of General Psychology,* 74 (April, 1966), 185-199.

CHAPTER 8

Abrams, Gene M. and N.S. Greenfield. *The New Hospital Psychiatry.* Proceedings of Interdisciplinary Conference sponsored by the University of Winsconsin Psychiatric Institute, June 5-7, 1969. New York: Academic Press, 1971.

Alexander, Leo. 'Limitations of experimentation on human beings with special reference to psychiatric patients,' *Diseases of the Nervous System,* 27 (July, 1966), 61-65.

Allport, Gordon W. *Personality and Social Encounter*. Boston: Beacon Press, 1960.

Appel, J.Z. 'Ethical and legal questions posed by recent advances in medicine,' *Journal of the American Medical Association,* 205 (August, 1968), 513-516.

Bakan, David. *Disease, Pain and Sacrifice*. Chicago: University of Chicago Press, 1968.

Baumeister, Alfred A. (ed.). *Mental Retardation: Appraisal, Education and Rehabilitation*. Chicago: Aldine Publishing Co., 1967.

Beech, H.R. *Changing Man's Behaviour*. London. Penguin Books, 1969.

Beecher, Henry K. *Research and the Individual: Human Studies*. Boston: Little, Brown and Co., 1970.

Beinaert, P. et al. (ed. P. Flood). *New Problems in Medical Ethics,* III. Westminster, Md.: Newman Press, 1956.

Bernstein, Norman R. (ed.). *Diminished People: Problems and Care of the Mentally Retarded*. Boston. Little, Brown and Co., 1970.

Bieber, Irving. *Homosexuality. A Psychoanalytic Study of the Male Homosexuals*. New York: Basic Books, 1963.

Borg, Gérard. *Le voyage à la drogue*. Paris: Editions Le Seuil, 1970.

Breggin, P.R. 'Psychotherapy as applied ethics,' *Psychiatry,* 34 (February, 1971), 59-74.

Brown, N.K. et al. 'The preservation of life,' *Journal of the American Medical Association,* 211 (January, 1970), 76-82.

Buckley, Michael J. *Morality and Homosexuality*. London: 1959.

Burton, Lloyd E. and Hugh H. Smith. *Public Health and Community Medicine*. Baltimore: Williams and Wilkins, 1970.

Carrera, Frank III, and P.L. Adams. 'An ethical perspective on operant conditioning,' *Journal of the American Academy of Child Psychiatry,* 9 (1970), 607-623.

Claridge, Gordon. *Drugs and Human Behaviour*. London: Penguin Books, 1970.

Corlis, R.B. and P. Rabe. *Psychotherapy from the Centre: A Humanistic View of Change and Growth*. Scranton: International Textbook, 1969.

Costello, Charles G. *Symptoms of Psychopathology*. New York: Wiley and Sons, 1970.

Curran, William J. 'Experimentation in children,' *Journal of the American Medical Association,* 210 (October, 1969), 77-83.

Curran, William J. 'Governmental regulation of the use of human subjects in medical research: the approach of two federal agencies,' Ethical Aspects of Experimentation with Human Subjects, *Daedalus* (Spring, 1969), 552-570.

Curran, William J., et al. 'Privacy, confidentiality and other legal considerations in the establishment of a centralized health-data system,' *New England Journal of Medicine,* 281 (July, 1969), 241-247.

Deuxième Congrès International de Morale Médicale. 2 vols. Paris: Ordre National des Médecins, 1966.

Epstein, Lynn C. and Louis Lasagna. 'Obtaining informed consent,' *Archives of Internal Medicine,* 123 (1969), 682-688.

Erikson, Erik H. *Insight and Responsibility*. Lectures on the ethical implications of psychoanalytic insight. New York: W.W. Norton, 1964.

Erikson, Erik H. 'Psychoanalysis and ongoing history: problems of identity, hatred and nonviolence,' *American Journal of Psychiatry*, 122 (September, 1965), 241-253.

Farber, Bernard. *Mental Retardation: Its Social Context and Social Consequences*. Boston: Houghton Mifflin Company, 1968.

Fletcher, John. 'Human experimentation: ethics in the consent situation,' *Law and Contemporary Problems*, 32 (1967), 620-649.

Flood, Peter. 'Narcoanalysis,' *New Problems in Medical Ethics, IV*. Cork: Mercier Press, 1963. 61-179.

Frankl, Viktor E. 'Beyond self-actualization and self-expression, *Psychiatry*, III (1962), 111-118.

Frankl, Viktor E. 'Beyond self-actualization and self-expression,' *Journal of Existential Psychiatry*, I (1960), 5-20.

Frankl, Viktor E. *The Doctor and the Soul*. New York: Knopf, 1965.

Frankl, Viktor E. 'Existential dynamics and neurotic escapism,' *Journal of Existential Psychiatry*, IV 1963), 27-42.

Frankl, Viktor E. *Man's Search for Meaning. An Introduction to Logotherapy*. London: Hodder and Stoughton, 1964.

Frankl, Viktor E. 'Paradoxical intention: a logotherapeutic technique,' *American Journal of Psychotherapy*, XIV (1960), 520-535.

Frankl, Viktor E. 'Psychiatry and man's quest for meaning,' *Journal of Religion and Health*, I (1962), 93-103.

Freund, Paul A. (comp.). *Experimentation with Human Subjects*. New York: G. Braziller, 1970.

Glasser, William. *Reality Therapy*. Los Angeles: Western Psychological Services, 1971.

Greenberg, Selig. *The Quality of Mercy: A Report on the Critical Condition of Hospital and Medical Care in America*. New York: Atheneum Publishers, 1971.

Grinspoon, Lester. *Marihuana Reconsidered*. Cambridge, Mass.: Harvard University Press, 1971.

Guttentag, Otto E. 'Ethical problems in human experimentation,' in *Ethical Issues in Medicine* (ed. E.F. Torrey). Boston: Little, Brown and Co., 1968. Pp. 195-226.

Hartmann, H. *Psychoanalysis and Moral Values*. New York: International Universities Press, 1960.

Johnson, Richard. *Existential Man: The Challenge of Psychotherapy*. Elmsford, N.Y.: Pergamon Press, 1971.

Jores, Arthur. *Vom kranken Menschen*. Stuttgart, 1960.

Knutson, A.L. 'Body transplants and ethical values,' *Social Science and Medicine*, 2 (1968-1969), 393-414.

Laurie, Peter. *Drugs*. London: Penguin Books, 1967.

London, Perry. *Modes and Morals of Psychotherapy*. New York: Holt, Rinehart, and Winston, 1964.

Lowe, C. Marshall. *Value Orientation in Counselling and Psychotherapy: The Meanings of Mental Health*. San Francisco: Chandler Publishing Co., 1969.

Margolis, Joseph. *Psychotherapy and Morality*. New York: Random House, 1965.

Mausner, Bernard and Ellen Platt. *Smoking: A Behavioral Analysis*. Elmsford, N.Y.: Pergamon Press, 1971.

McNeil, J.N. et al. 'Community psychiatry and ethics,' *American Journal of Orthopsychiatry*, 40 (January, 1970), 22-29.

Menninger, Karl. 'The new violence and the new psychiatry,' *Bulletin of the Menninger Clinic*, 32 (1968), 341-354.

Menolascino, Frank J. (ed.). *Psychiatric Approaches to Mental Retardation*. New York: Basic Books, 1970.

Merlis, Sidney (ed.). *Non-Scientific Constraints on Medical Research*. New York: Raven Press, 1970.

Milbauer, Barbara. *Drug Abuse and Addiction*. New York: Crown Publishers, 1970.

O'Connor, Elizabeth. *Our Many Selves*. New York: Harper and Row, 1971.

Oursler, Will. *The Healing Power of Faith*. Kingswood (Surrey), 1958.

Page, Irving R. 'The ethics of heart transplantation,' *Journal of the American Medical Association*, 207 (January, 1969), 109-113.

Pappworth, M.H. *Human Guinea Pigs: Experimentation on Man*. Boston: Beacon Press, 1968.

Pastorelli, Fr. *Servitude et grandeur de la maladie*. Paris, 1967.

Plante, Marcus L. 'An analysis of informed consent,' *Fordham Law Review*, 36 (May, 1968), 639-672.

Protection of the Individual as a Research Subject. Washington, D.C.: Public Health Service. December 12, 1966.

Ruitenbeek, Hendrik M. *Group Therapy Today: Styles, Methods and Techniques*. Los Angeles: Western Psychological Services, 1970.

Sarason, Seymour B. and John Doris. *Psychological Problems in Mental Deficiency*. (4th ed.) New York: Harper and Row, 1969.

Smith, Robert M. *An Introduction to Mental Retardation*. New York: McGraw-Hill Book Company, 1971.

Stern, E. Mark and Bert G. Marino. *Psychotheology*. New York: Newman Press, 1970.

Stevens, Rosemary. *American Medicine and the Public Interest*. New Haven: Yale University Press, 1971.

Szasz, T.S. *The Ethics of Psychoanalysis: The Theory and Method of Autonomous Psychotherapy*. New York: Basic Books, 1965.

Tweedie, Donold F. *The Christian and the Couch. An Introduction to Christian Logotherapy*. Grand Rapids, Mich.: Baker House, 1963.

Vadenberg, J.H. *The Psychology of the Sickbed*. Penn.: Duquesne University Press, 1966.

Westman, Wesley C. *Drug Epidemic*. New York: Dial Press, 1970.

Wilkinson, Rupert. *The Prevention of Drinking Problems: Alcohol Control and Cultural Influences*. New York: Oxford University Press, 1970.

World Medical Association. 'Declaration of Helsinki: Recommendations Guiding Doctors in Clinical Research,' *World Medical Journal*, 11 (1964), 281.

ANALYTICAL INDEX

breakthrough: 132, 172
breast-feeding: 62
brotherhood: 12, 69, 98, 215

call(ing): 43, 45-46, 65-68, 180, 200, 207
cancer: 27, 128, 190
Cannabis: see marijuana
Capetown: 135
Casti Connubii: 9, 47, 105, 115
casuistry: 19, 62, 100, 109, 127
cell: 19, 51, 77, 79-80, 83, 86, 93
cerebral cortex: see cortex
chemistry: 60, 62, 89
child: 39-40, 73-74, 78, 83, 91, 93-94, 98, 108, 110-111, 114, 117-118, 153, 158, 168, 188, 195, 216-217
childbirth: 199, 205-206
Christian Science: xii, 145, 149
chromosomes: 18, 63-64, 187
Church: 2-3, 8-9, 16-17, 35-36, 38, 71, 76, 88, 90-91, 95-96, 100, 103-104, 106, 115, 116-119, 121, 132, 156, 193-194
Church in the Modern World: 8, 76, 88
code: ethical: 17, 20, 23-41, 209, 212, 214
code: genetic: 52, 77, 80, 83
coma: 135
commitment: 24, 125-126, 156-157, 195-196
common good: 16, 21, 69, 117-118, 201
communication: 32, 46, 52, 78, 130-131, 163, 170, 196, 202, 214
Communism: 33, 190
community: 4-6, 12, 16, 24, 28, 36, 45, 51, 61, 63, 67, 71, 143, 152-153, 192, 196, 198, 201, 213
compassion: 27, 145, 161, 164, 166
competence: 17, 19, 28, 35, 74, 85, 87, 89-90, 125, 132, 142, 163, 171, 179, 182, 188, 192, 196, 213-214
complex: 69, 93, 161, 178

complexity: 19, 57, 78, 84, 87, 89, 163
compulsion: 70-71, 175
computer: 52-53
conception: 1, 33, 75-76, 85-86, 97, 114, 155
condition: 1-2, 7, 15, 36, 39, 52, 82, 84, 93, 97, 108, 125, 128-130, 141-142, 148-149, 152, 154-155, 168, 174, 180, 185, 191, 194, 196, 199, 201-203, 212, 214-217
condom: 92
confidence: 26, 65, 71, 126, 199, 201-203, 205
conflict: xii, 38, 42, 84, 101, 102, 168, 187-188, 193, 195
conjugal: 88, 105, 189, 206
conscience: 9, 17, 25, 29, 32, 35-39, 41, 71, 85, 89, 102, 105, 113, 115-118, 158, 169, 179-181, 209
conscious(ness): xiii, 13, 18, 46, 50-52, 61, 73, 80, 82-83, 111, 125-126, 132-133, 138, 142, 169, 172-174, 176, 178, 182, 206-207, 216-217
consent: 40, 182, 211, 215-217
contraception: 85-86, 88, 99, 102, 104-106, 150
contribution: 6, 11, 13, 57, 69, 74, 94-95, 107, 112, 173, 196, 199
control: 24, 149, 162, 182, 185-187, 191, 204
conversion: xi, 112, 164, 186, 189
cooperation: 15, 30, 34-35, 40, 75, 89, 97, 145, 153, 166, 171, 179, 183, 216
co-responsibility: 10, 34, 59, 73
corpse: 51, 63
cortex: 18, 50, 52, 77, 81-85, 86, 132-134, 140, 159
cosmos: 21, 44, 54
counselling: 19, 89, 112-115, 181, 184
covenant: 45, 166, 199, 200-201, 204-205
creation: 1, 12, 43-45, 62, 124, 158, 164, 172, 208

237

238

239

Q

240

241

242

243

245

247

NAME INDEX

Adam, 44
Adler, A., 173
Aesculapius, 32
Albert the Great (St), 76
Aldrich, C.K., 130
Alexandre, 135
Allport, G.W., 174, 178
Alphonsus Liguori (St), 103, 113
Apollo, 32
Aquinas, Thomas (St), 9, 46, 47, 55, 76
Aristotle, xii, 9, 46, 47
Arnoldt, R., 201
Augustine (St), 47, 99

Babinet, P., 132
Baltzell, W.H., 128
Beecher, H.K., 135
Bernhart, J., 156
Bieber, I., 187, 188
Binding, K., 144
Böckle, F., 81, 95
Bolech, P., 160
Boone, W.J., 140
Boros, L., 124
Brewer, L.A., 133
Brim, O.G., 130
Buber, M., 46
Buckley, M.J., 186, 188
Bulger, R.J., 127

Callahan, D., 95
Camus, 195
Casper, B., 136
Chiavacci, E., 81, 93
Claridge, G., 190
Conley, J.C., 128
Crespy, G., 166
Curran, C., 46

Davidson, H.A., 202
De Chardin, Teilhard, 82, 110, 172
Decourt, J., 188
De Martel, 183
Donceel, J.F., 95
Dostoievsky, 70

Dubost, C., 138
Durand-Dassier, J., 198

Ebner, F., 46
Entralgo, P.L., 28
Erikson, E., 160, 196
Eve, 44

Fishgold, H., 134
Fleckenstein, H., 160
Flood, P., 118
Fourrier, xiii
Francis of Assisi (St), 47
Francoeur, T., 94
Frankl, V., 48, 49, 167, 169, 173, 174, 175, 176, 177, 178, 179, 180
Freud, S., xii, 172, 173, 174, 175, 176, 177

Galileo, 8
Gastgeber, K., 157
Giesen, D., 91
Glees, P., 81
Goulon, M., 132
Gregory XIV, 100
Gründel, J., 95
Guinet, P., 188
Guirdham, A., 160
Gustafson, J.M., 102, 112, 113, 114
Gütgemann, A., 140

Häring, B., 75, 85, 114
Heidegger, M., 48
Hellegers, A.E., 79, 80, 95
Heraclitus, 47
Hildegard (St), 156
Hippocrates, xi, xii, 21, 26, 32, 33, 54, 61
Hitler, A., 30, 142, 144, 150
Hoche, A., 144
Holzman, 111
Husserl, E., 7
Huxley, A., 62

Jerome (St), 99
John of the Cross, (St), 156

249

250